Inside Group Work

Inside Group Work

Fiona McDermott

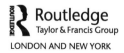

Routledge
Taylor & Francis Group
LONDON AND NEW YORK

First published 2002 by Allen & Unwin

Published 2020 by Routledge
2 Park Square, Milton Park, Abingdon, Oxon OX14 4RN
605 Third Avenue, New York, NY 10017

Routledge is an imprint of the Taylor & Francis Group, an informa business

National Library of Australia
Cataloguing-in-Publication entry:

McDermott, Fiona, 1951- .
    Inside group work: a guide to reflective practice.

    Bibliography.
    Includes Index

    1. Group facilitation. 2. Social groups. 3. Teams in the workplace. I. Title.
    158.2

Set in 10.5/14 ACaslon Regular by Midland Typesetters

ISBN-13: 9781865088921 (pbk)

CONTENTS

ACKNOWLEDGMENTS

In developing this book, I held conversations with the following people, some of whom are participants in groups, some of whom lead or facilitate groups, and some of whom do both: Bernard; Breast Cancer Therapy Group; Bob Pease; Bridget Roberts; Chris Laming; Cynthia Holland; Helen Lee; Lou Harms; Robyn Chellew; Maria Rossi; Janet Spink.

Their contribution has been extremely valuable, playing a central role in this book. I thank them most sincerely.

During 2001, I 'workshopped' parts of this book with students taking the Social Work Practice with Groups subject in the Bachelor of Social Work program at the University of Melbourne. Their feedback and responses to some of the material presented have been very useful. I thank them for their enthusiastic engagement with many of the ideas in the book and their assistance in refining aspects of it.

My co-facilitator of seventeen years' group work practice, Christine Hill, remains an invaluable source of support and critique. Her comments on Chapter 9 were most useful and constructive. Associate Professor Wendy Weeks gave generous and helpful comments on Chapter 3.

I also wish to acknowledge my colleagues in the School of Social Work at the University of Melbourne, and Elizabeth Weiss at Allen & Unwin for her always helpful editorial comments.

INTRODUCTION

A book about working with groups confronts us with a dilemma: can we really learn about something as dynamic and interactive as group work from the static medium of a book? Here is what a group participant and a group worker say:

> You have to have done a bit (of group work) yourself to understand the process. I think it's not something you could learn from a textbook or have someone tell you or take down notes at a lecture—I think you would have to have experienced [it] yourself in a personal way, not experienced it by sitting in and observing a group functioning but you being a participating member of a group. If you haven't done that I don't think you could effectively lead a group . . . because you just couldn't understand what it was like for people who were in the group. (Bernard, a participant in a psychotherapy group)

> If you want to work with groups—be in a few of them . . . find a group that is doing something that is of relevance to you and

during the years you're [studying], be in this group as well because you will learn far more from [a course in group work] if you have that experience. (Helen Lee, social action group leader and member)

These two comments pose a challenge: how can a book about group work practice compete with the powerful impact of personal experience in understanding and learning group work? While there is no substitute for actually gaining personal experience by participating in a group, it is equally difficult to avoid experience with groups—they are everywhere and there's no escaping them! We are born into a group, grow up in one, are educated and socialised into groups, worship, work and play in groups, marry into groups, die as members of groups—some people even have sex in groups. So-called 'reality TV' with shows like *Big Brother*, *Survivor*, *The Mole* and *Castaway 2000* play on our fascination with the ways groups work, with observing and empathising with the vicissitudes of 'insiders' and 'outsiders'.

It can be quite surprising to count the number of groups we belong to, or that we acknowledge as significant to us in some way, to discover just how many there are. Although I do not consider myself to be a particularly 'groupy' kind of person, I calculate that there are at least twelve groups to which I currently belong. It is equally interesting and informative to list the groups which are anathema to us and with which we avoid forming any connections. And to further identify those groups which we do not formally belong to, but which we recognise as influencing us—for example, the World Health Organization—increases the number of groups impacting on our lives quite significantly. In fact, the very ubiquity of groups makes them almost invisible, like the air we breathe and the sounds we hear. Yet, just as air and sound are central to our existence, groups as a form of personal and social organisation play a vital and influential role (for good as well as ill) in affecting the course of our lives.

This book is intended to complement and build on what we

already know from everyday life about groups, and in so doing to provide some assistance to beginning group workers who want to set up and lead or facilitate groups, as well as those who want to extend their knowledge and understanding of group work practice. It is intended as a guide to thinking about groups, about what we do in and with them. In order to make the best possible uses of groups, we need to understand what happens when a collection of individuals get together.

Why work with groups?

Social workers, psychologists, community workers, youth workers and other service providers in the human services field spend much of their time working with groups—as staff members, as colleagues—using groups as intervention strategies. While research findings on the effectiveness of group work are limited in scope and volume (see Rose and Feldman 1987; Tindale et al. 1998; Corey 2000), many of us believe that working collectively with colleagues, fellow service providers and service users can be extremely productive, helpful and enjoyable. However, it can also be a source of stress and tension. Some groups never gel, others are riddled with conflict, and some just fall away. But there are always other stories of groups that flourish and prosper, of groups and group members who achieve unexpectedly positive outcomes, and of groups that become rich sources of social capital and fully realised citizenship. Working with groups has been, and remains, a vital part of the practice of many human service professionals. Papell's comments (1997, p. 11) with regard to the history of group work practice in social work capture well the experience of many human service professions. She notes that its history reflects 'the essentials of the human condition—mutual aid and caritas, relationships, helping, sharing, play and work, social concern, collective action, empowerment, survival'.

In this book, our focus is on the work social workers, youth workers, community workers and other professionals do through the medium of group work in order to achieve outcomes that further the interests and needs of group participants. Group participants may be experiencing problems related to illness or disability, they may be the object of stigma or marginalisation such as those who experience psychiatric disability, or the conditions of their lives may have denied them opportunities for personal development and self-fulfillment. Other groups, such as community development and social action groups, form in order to bring about social or structural change (and sometimes to prevent change) through collective effort. Throughout this book, group workers and participants—the 'insiders'—speak about their understanding of their work, the kind of group they facilitate or belong to, and the structures and processes which characterise their group. Their experience of collective work, and the structures and processes which facilitate this, contribute to our understanding of group work.

Working with groups, whether as group leader or organiser, or as group participant, provides opportunities to achieve outcomes that are frequently impossible or inappropriate to reach in any other way. While not all groups operate on completely democratic or collective premises, the potential to challenge the status quo within groups is often both possible and encouraged. The group comprises resources and strengths that no one individual can provide for him/herself. Indeed, the group can become something of a free market economy in which individuals may contribute and resource themselves and others in a reciprocal and mutually beneficial way.

Defining a group

In the process of counting the groups to which we belong (or which we avoid), or which we acknowledge as significant to us in some way, we have to define what a group is. There are several ways we might do this. We might identify the group as *geographical*—for example, made up of residents of the street we live in, or the country we reside in. Or we might identify the group as being made up of people with *a shared interest*—for example, a book discussion group. The group may be an *institution* such as a church or a school. It may comprise people with a *shared political or social perspective*, such as a disability rights group. It may be a *work- or task-focused* group such as a group within the organisation where we work or, for example, the second-hand clothing shop where we volunteer our services. Our definition may have a more *subjective* element to it such as when we see our friends as comprising a group to which we belong. Or it may be a group which contributes to our *sense of identity*, such as our family or an ethnic group.

The moment we try to define what precisely we mean by a group, we are in difficulty. Is it a case of numbers, or shared interests, or differences, or shared experiences or temporality? Is it all of these things or none of them? Are those we communicate with on the internet a group? Is a group a thing or an experience? How do we distinguish, for example, between a group and a football crowd, or a group and an audience at the opera, or a group and a gang? When girl gang members were asked by researchers to distinguish between their peer group and a gang, the majority could not do so. One young woman said: '[The gang] is like a second family. Because I don't have my dad, I know my homeboys are there for me . . . and always will be 'cause that's just the way it is.' (Petersen 2000, p. 145) When the young women gang members were encouraged to elaborate, they did discuss the elements of violence and criminal activity which academics and researchers have included in their definition of what a gang is; however, left to themselves, a gang and a peer group were more or less synonymous to 'insiders'.

Until we define a situation, it is very difficult to know how to act or 'be' in that situation. In order to do so, we need to accommodate, or 'frame' (Goffman 1974), a situation to be a particular kind of situation. Once we have framed it, we have invested it with meaning. By investing it with meaning, we are able to know how to act and what to do in that situation—what ways of thinking or acting are appropriate or inappropriate. So how we frame something makes a crucial difference to how we perceive, interpret and understand phenomena and experiences. In framing something *as* something, we are marking boundaries or imposing borders, indicating what is 'inside' and what is 'outside'. However, simultaneously we are contextualising these experiences or phenomena because the frame we impose is an attempt to limit and define this perceptual field in relation to the context in which it is occurring. McLachlan and Reid (1994, p. 54) comment: 'frames function both as part of the structure of what they enclose . . . and part of the "outside" world against which the enclosed text or activity is framed'. To frame an activity or an experience as a 'group' is to set up expectations about the kinds of things that might happen, the kind of attention or action that might be required of participants. Very importantly, it will affect what kinds of interpretations are made about 'what is happening here', 'what it means', and 'how it came to mean this'.

Many people have defined groups. Shaw (1981, p. 454), for example, offers a somewhat minimal definition, proposing that a group is: 'two or more people who are interacting with one another in such a manner that each person influences and is influenced by each person'. Forsyth (1999) samples the prevailing definitions of groups and notes what others in the field have identified as the central features of groups. These include:

- communication;
- influence;
- interaction and a sense of 'we-ness';
- interdependence;
- interrelations;
- psychological significance;
- shared identity;
- structure—the group as a social unit with status, roles, values and norms.

This suggests that groups are characterised by at least two persons, shared space and shared purpose. The interactions taking place amongst members may be important in the development of common goals, norms and roles, and some sense of belonging. Within the context of a group, participants find the possibility of making comparisons between themselves and others, which can become an influential source of control and reward for members. As such, groups may play a part in defining the individual's sense of reality. While groups are extremely powerful phenomena, they also hold the possibility of learning how to share that power.

Each of these definitions has its usefulness and its limitations. Indeed, the moment we attempt to capture what a group is, we place a boundary around those elements which are *in* and hence comprise the group, and those which are *out* and thereby become part of the group's boundary.

The notion of the group as a *bounded social experience* of some kind is useful in conveying the somewhat arbitrary nature of naming and framing whatever it is we call a group. Two further elements are important. Firstly, members of groups communicate in some way to one another. Secondly, the experience of being in a group needs to be acknowledged by participants both subjectively (a sense of belonging, however slight) and objectively (to something that exists in some kind of tangible form, recognisable to themselves and others). Indeed, the group can be thought of as exemplifying a particular mode of human interaction. Groups generate interaction that is different from, for example, one-to-one conversations. They thus create a different kind of experience and a different 'level' of being.

What are we studying when we study groups?

In the first instance, when we study human groups we are studying a central and primary part of the constitution of social reality. Here, within a variety of group or collective experiences, our sense of identity—of self, of social citizenship—is recognised and expressed.

We can also interpret the actions of people working collectively in many different ways, some of which may occur simultaneously. Groups exemplify:

- sets of interactions;
- sets of power relations;
- a particular kind of social and individual discourse that is different from that which occurs between one individual and another;
- a site where individuals' desires and fears interplay as they react and respond to the threats and anxieties which the intimacy of a group conjures up;
- a site where there is interplay and struggle between various interpretations of social reality for legitimacy, acceptance and ascendancy;
- an aspect of social (actual) reality and of individual fantasy. The individual and other group participants interact and create a social experience both in the 'here and now' as well as in their own minds, in the fantasies and imaginings that infuse and colour their interpretations of what is happening;
- the individual meanings which people give to their intersubjective experience. Within the group context we can study the language and the metaphors people use to communicate and share their experiences with one another. It is a particular kind of discourse that becomes available for us to understand and enter, however partially, the social and experiential world of participants.

These ways of describing what is available for us to observe in groups only hint at the enormous variety and richness which may emerge out of collaborative work. It is the task of the group worker and group participants to maximise this potential.

Organisation of this book

This book emerged from two sources: my own practice as a group worker in a variety of settings, and my group work teaching with social work students. One of the principal challenges my practice and teaching experience generated was how to infuse the teaching of group work concepts and skills with the richness and complexity of 'real life' work with groups. Too often, group work teaching can become formulaic and banal, even with a modicum of experiential learning opportunities. My solution has been to turn to a number of group leaders and participants for help.

I began my research for this book by talking with group leaders and participants. Our conversations were wide-ranging and thought-provoking. From these conversations I have selected comments which illustrate many of the points made in the book with the 'real life' experience of those who know best what group work is all about. While the freshness and originality of many of these comments may not completely compensate for being in a group oneself, they do give us the opportunity to think about our experience with groups, how we might come to understand it and use it better.

The book begins (Chapter 2) by introducing the people to whom I spoke in preparing the text. They comprise a mix of group leaders and group participants working from a range of theoretical positions, with various types of groups and differing purposes for working collectively. This range is indicative of the variety of work in the field and the eclecticism of group work practice.

Chapter 3 provides a theoretical guide through this eclecticism. It is a key chapter in arguing that firm theoretical grounding for group work is essential in ensuring practice which is critical and reflective. Drawing on prevalent perspectives in the field, five vantage points for theorising group work practice are presented. Each of these perspectives proceeds from a central image or metaphor for what a group is—a power base, a system, a container of individuals, a container of properties, a site for meaning construction. Current theoretical debates, in particular the developments in critical postmodern theory, are explored in relation to the interconnections between these various theoretical perspectives.

The next three chapters address the complex issue of group leadership. The argument is made that leadership is a resource which all group participants contribute to and share in. Leadership refers to the possibility of influencing the way the group works. The power that is synonymous with leading a group emerges from the reciprocity of relationships in the group. Power itself is a resource rather than a given. It is expressed through the resources which all participants bring to the group. These resources comprise knowledge, experience, structural positioning, personal characteristics and capabilities. Rather than providing a list of abstract 'leadership skills', Chapter 5 explores the par ticular kind of capability that is indispensable to group leaders—that of 'thinking group'. 'Thinking group' refers to the capacity to approach the group as a whole, with a mental and cognitive frame or schema for working that encompasses everything that happens within the group. In order to 'think group', workers and participants need to be receptive to the metaphors and images that are created in the collective encounter of a number of individuals. This requires that they be skilled participant–observers, listeners and thinkers who keep in mind and remember what has gone before in the group and who are attuned to accommodating information from both the internal and external context in which the group exists. How they speak and what they say in the group reflects the interpretations that emerge from participating and observing, listening, thinking and remembering. This is discussed in Chapter 6.

Chapter 7 focuses on the formation of a group, what type of group it is, who is in it and what structures will be adopted. To form and structure a group means to make decisions about the boundaries which are to be drawn around the group. These decisions clearly relate both to the theoretical basis from which the group derives and the purpose which it is to serve. They include such things as whether the group is to be open or closed, time-limited or time-unlimited, homogenous or heterogenous, and what activities it will undertake.

Chapter 8 explores the 'life' of the group. An argument is put that time is a central organising principle for group work. What happens to the group over time—what changes, what occurs, what does not happen, what is achieved—depends on the time available and how group participants make use of their time. Time-limited groups are discussed in relation to the stages and phases that describe their likely progress, while time-unlimited groups which have a different temporal perspective are discussed in relation to the way in which their progress may be understood.

Chapter 9 provides a description and analysis of 'critical issues' in the life of a group. The choice of particular issues has been made in relation to those most frequently raised by the people I spoke with, or those which have been noted by writers in the group work literature. We will look at the first meeting, the arrival of a new member, conflict, a decision to leave, and the final meeting of a group. Examples are drawn from a range of groups—social action, psychotherapy, support, psychoeducational.

The final chapter looks at what is meant by a 'good' group, or 'good' group work practice. The central point made in this chapter is that the group itself exemplifies research-in-action as participants cycle back and forward, observing and reflecting on their progress. This dynamism and vitality makes researching and evaluating groups difficult. However, various ways of recording and reflecting on the group are identified as providing ways to monitor the group's progress. They may also form the basis for developing theoretical and practice-based knowledge about group work.

Theoretical base

The theoretical base underlying this book derives from a social constructionist perspective in which the group is framed as a site of

11

meaning construction. This includes recognition that the meaning one makes of the work of a group always refers to the context in which it is embedded. This context is temporal and historical. The group is identified as constituting, and as a constituent part of, the social world. Working from this frame of reference allows the group worker to simultaneously attend to, and make use of, knowledge referring to the structural organisation of the social world, the material conditions of participants, and the emotional and experienced 'inner' world of the group.

But what is the context within which we are thinking about the practice of group work? Here at the beginning of the twenty-first century we are confronted by the contradictions posed and imposed by the forces of globalisation. On the one hand, we encounter the dissolution of economic boundaries and the erosion of cultural difference through the impact of mass communication and information networks. On the other hand, we recognise the increasing emergence of groups and communities asserting their difference and separateness in a bid to maintain a sense of identity and to establish themselves as sites of resistance. These two contradictory forces seem to be on a collision course. The greater the impact of globalisation and mass culture, the greater the likelihood that such identity-focused groups will become more inward-looking and, in the process, authoritarian and coercive in striving to draw their boundaries ever more stringently against the impact of globalisation. However, this 'horizontal society' (see Friedman 1999) in which there is weakening of the authority of parental or governmental or institutional forces in favour of the influence of identity groups based on, for example, race, gender or religion, also has the potential to foster social cohesion.

Given these prevailing conditions, we are confronted with questions about how social cohesion, which makes collective life possible, can be attained and retained. The contemporary social, political and economic context is one characterised by potentially overwhelming change, anxiety and uncertainty (Giddens 1991). Beck

(1986) has described it as living in the 'risk society', vulnerable to disasters on a global scale. In surveying this contemporary scene, Touraine (2000, p. 13) poses the question: 'can we live together, or will we allow ourselves to be reduced to the status of passive consumers of a mass culture produced by a globalized economy?'

Current debates have addressed these issues with reference to the concept of social capital. While definitions of social capital are contested, Cox and Caldwell (2000, p. 50) note that the concept refers to the linkages amongst people which 'sustain mutuality and the capacity to resolve the conflicts and tensions associated with change'. Social capital can most easily be identified when it enables people, organisations, communities and nations to work collaboratively, respect values and differences, and resolve disputes by going beyond sectional interests in search of the common good (2000, p. 59). Trust lies at the basis of such endeavours which require vigilant and constant opposition to the emergence of prejudice and exploitation. Or, as Lyons (2000, p. 168) defines it: 'Social capital is the mechanism that enables people to trust one another sufficiently to work collectively, to solve common pool resource problems.' Very importantly, it cannot be said to be social capital if this connectedness and cohesion are derived from practices which exclude or demonise 'others' outside the group (Cox and Caldwell 2000, p. 59).

Putnam (1995, 2000) has argued that social capital is what makes democracies work. However, his research (and that of others—see Winter 2000; Hogan and Owen 2000) has indicated that its stocks are in decline. Measures of social capital derive from evidence throughout the last decade of a decline in participation rates in voluntary work and active membership of voluntary organisations, as well as participation in political action. We know from research in many fields, but particularly in health and mental health (see Warner 1994; Walsh 1994; Willie et al. 1995; Baum et al. 2000), that social isolation and exclusion are bad for us. Indeed, the comments noted in this book from group workers and participants frequently underscore the emotional and physical well-being that group participation brings, not to mention the sense of empowerment that success in achieving tangible outcomes delivers.

Working with groups pulls us headlong into the contradictions of contemporary globalised life. But our understanding of this context also presents us with challenges. The tendency towards an isolating and inward-looking group work is ever present if we react only to the uncertainties, anxieties and turbulence of everyday (globalised) life. However, within the group itself there are opportunities to enable ourselves and others to develop our capacities as actors. Through dialogue and collaboration with others, we can move towards establishing the coherence of our individual life stories, which counteracts the incoherence and discontinuities which surround us. Working in and with groups can be a significant means of strengthening individuals as well as building social capital. As Giddens (1991, p. 2) points out: 'No matter how local their specific contexts of action, individuals contribute to and directly promote social influences that are global in their consequences and implications.' This means that those of us who work with and in groups are positioned to enhance the accumulation of social capital.

Group work is about building bonds between people which depend on the establishment of trusting relationships. It is also about helping to forge connections between people who may be different or unlike one another. This latter activity—finding common ground across differences—is the more difficult, and it is here that group workers and participants require knowledge and skills. Essential to this is the capability required to assist participants in dealing with conflict and in accepting 'outsiders'. In this way, relationships may become truly reciprocal. Furthermore, the trust, cohesion and reciprocity enacted within the small group (be it psychotherapeutic, psychoeducational, support, self-help or social action) must be transferred to the 'wider' world outside. Through that process, group participation can contribute to the social capital available for all of us. Seeing the place of group work from this position enables us to think about and construct new forms of personal and collective life which do not succumb to the authoritarian and introverted structures prompted by globalisation. Group work, then, has a potentially vital role to play in the personal, social and political world—but only if it is a group work which recognises itself as occurring within and shaping that context.

2

GROUP PURPOSE:
'Why would you do it on your own?'

So Helen, what was your purpose in setting up the group?
Why would you do it on your own? Fundamental to any social change or addressing social injustice is solidarity. You have to get together with other people because . . . [the] baseline is a commitment to democracy . . . to do that you need to connect with other people who are also affected and listen to them and their perspective and work out how you can come to some common ground because . . . one voice on its own is not going to achieve much.

Social change, addressing injustice, solidarity, democracy, connection, listening, finding common ground, achieving goals—in replying to my question, Helen Lee easily identified eight purposes for her group, each of them almost sufficient on its own to justify the group's existence. Furthermore, her answer strongly asserts that the decision to form a group comes out of her recognition that a group is the best way to achieve these purposes—in a sense, from her perspective, there is no question to answer.

While Helen is referring to a social action group, similar senti-
ments are expressed by leaders and participants across the range of
groups—psychotherapy, psychoeducation, support, advocacy, self-help.
For all of them, there is something of particular value that emerges
through the collaboration of minds and bodies in a group that cannot
be achieved in any other way. In this and subsequent chapters, we will
hear how other group leaders and participants have answered this
question. They talk about their experiences, beliefs and theories about
groups—about why they don't want to do what they do on their own.
I met with each of them in coffee bars, offices and around kitchen
tables. In our conversations we shared stories and anecdotes, swapping
those ideas and understandings captured through experience. Snatches
of these conversations accompany our progress through this book. But
to begin with, we need to know who is talking and what they are
talking about.

Helen Lee: we met in her large and rambling inner-city house. Our
conversation was accompanied by tweeting birds, children coming
and going, and contented gurgles from her newborn daughter. Amidst
all the busyness of her life, Helen has been involved in many different
groups. The one she chose to talk about was a social action group set
up to prevent the closure of a community medical service—an
outcome the group successfully achieved.

It was really clear that [the proposed closure] was what the group
was for . . . the issue was very clear cut and something people felt
strongly about . . . it was very much a group with a purpose and it
brought people together.

Bernard: we met at his club in the city over lunch. For several
months he has been in an ongoing psychoanalytically oriented psychotherapy group which meets every day for one hour. Previously,
Bernard was in the same group for a period of eighteen months. He
calls it an *analytic group* and describes its purpose as:

To understand yourself better. You'll do that best in therapy if what you bring in are things about yourself that you don't understand or that to you seem irrational. That's why [the leader] encourages people to bring in dreams because they're your own creation and they give a clue to things about you.

On a warm sunny early spring day, I drove to country Victoria to meet with *Chris Laming*. After recent rain, the countryside was green and lush with soft hills and blue sky. The economic picture for this region however, is less attractive—high unemployment, the highest rate of domestic violence in the state, extensive public housing and poverty in the small towns along the highway. At the community health centre Chris has developed a group program for men who are violent. The program offers an open group and a closed, structured twelve-week program which participants move into from the open group. Chris describes the purpose of the group as:

about listening, about supporting, about challenging men to change behaviours that are clearly identified as abusive . . . having a common space where they can put their stuff and get something back—a sense that 'I'm not alone, I'm not the only one in this mess. I can do something about it.'

Robyn Chellew has been a community health social worker for many years, as well as finding time for developing her own private counselling practice. Her work has included both family counselling and group work in which she has developed her special interest in step-family and teenage parent education programs. Robyn brings this wide-ranging experience to her teaching of group work to social work students. Between classes we met for lunch to talk about one of the groups she had most recently established. It is a psychoeducational group for step-families comprising couples coming to talk about issues about building their families and how to work together as a family and build a sense of family. The purpose of this group is:

> to teach couples about what it is that is different about step-families . . . To educate them about how children feel about step-families, based on research . . . giving them skills and tools to understand what they're observing, and to normalise those feelings and hopefully give them skills to handle [the situation].

Cynthia Holland is a polymath—social worker, lawyer, artist, teacher, medical researcher. Presently she works in the gynaeoncology unit of a large public hospital. Her group work is with mothers and children where the mothers are going through cancer treatment or sometimes consequential palliative care. The group she has developed allows her to draw on her artistic and imaginative talents, using painting, drawing, modelling and playing with the children and their mothers. The purpose of Cynthia's group is:

> to commemorate [the children's lives] with mother together . . . a specialty relationship between the child and mum. It's about the uniqueness of their relationship with mum, individualised yet shared with other members [of the group]. You're trying to equip them with hope of a future family life, based on the model they've shared.

Bob Pease and I began our conversation in the busy cafeteria of the city university campus where he teaches. Before long, the noise and clattering dishes move us to the quiet of a teaching room. Bob established Men Against Sexual Assault more than a decade ago as both a social action and a consciousness-raising group. This twofold purpose is not always an easy alliance, but Bob argues that:

the men's group is a space that affirms the kind of masculine subjectivity that's not affirmed in other places. There's an affirmation that this is a valuable subjectivity we're trying to construct with each other ... I can have particular kinds of conversations with this group that I just can't have very easily with other men ... we need to do things collectively, not individually, because we want to be political in the world.

Each time I have attended performances by the Women's Circus, I have been captivated by the skill and energy of the performers, the movement and imaginative formations of the women's bodies working as an ensemble. It is a group which needs an audience, not only to enjoy and be uplifted by the colour and light of the show but for performers themselves to demonstrate their outward-looking, forward-moving focus. I spoke with *Bridget Roberts*, a member of the Circus. She describes the Women's Circus as:

a community physical theatre group ... It's set up with very clear aims from the beginning—to do performance in a feminist way ... the fundamental aim is to help women regain a sense of control over our bodies and the first priority group for women [in asking to join the Circus] are those who are survivors of sexual abuse ... It's meeting to do things around a common purpose, and it's the purpose that unites and includes women ...

Lou Harms has worked with a wide range of groups. Now a lecturer in the School of Social Work, she teaches group work as well as other subjects in the curriculum. For many years she has co-led a psychoeducational/psychotherapeutic group focused around positive ageing. This group has an unusual structure. Auspiced by a large city church, the group may comprise as many as 80 participants who meet throughout one day. The group is structured to combine large and small group discussion with input and challenge provided by Lou's co-leader, the founder of the group. Lou describes the group's purpose as 'putting the issues of positive ageing into a psychological context'. People come together in the group 'with the explicit purpose of sharing experience'.

The use of focus groups in research is becoming an increasingly frequent occurrence, but one which does not always recognise that considerable group work skills are required to maximise the potential of this method. *Janet Spink*, a social worker with experience in working with individuals, families and groups, as well as having an extensive research background, was ideally placed to discuss her work with focus groups. In the weeks prior to our meeting, Janet had conducted eighteen focus groups as part of her current research work. The purpose of focus groups, she noted, was to gather research data within a tight time-frame, where access to a number of people at one time was required, and where the process of developing ideas was valued. However, this may not always be the same purpose participants hold. In relation to the health issues she was using focus groups to explore, Janet commented:

I had to find some way of acknowledging their pain which didn't engage with it too deeply, because that was not what you were there for . . . people are talking about their own experience, thinking they might die, or their experience of having a baby . . . so in some ways the focus groups are debriefing [for participants] whereas that's not the purpose of the group.

Maria Rossi invited me to meet at her home on a hot pre-Christmas Saturday, making time amid her family and self-help group commitments for our conversation. She is a founding member of a self-help and advocacy group concerned with fertility issues, weathering conflict and high personal demands as she works to bring the vision she shares with others towards fulfilment. Maria is emphatic about what drives her to be part of this group: 'For me it's a cause—I want to change the way people see [this issue] and that's all I want to do!' Maria identifies two purposes as central to her group:

Children don't have a say. It's great if their parents can be equipped to deal with the issues . . . so for me there are two things which become important: the consumer advocacy—we advocate only for children—and education. One of my dreams is to actually have an education program before parents have their children which allows them to really understand things and so they could decide if they really wanted to do it [become pregnant].

Heather Clarke is passionate about her interest in and commitment to working with women. As a social worker in a community health centre (and in collaboration with her co-facilitator, a community health nurse), she saw that the formation of a group with the dual purposes of providing support and increasing participants' understanding of issues affecting their emotional and mental health was needed. Heather drew from her practice experience:

I was seeing a lot of women who seemed to be presenting very similar sorts of issues around needing to start to care for themselves in their lives: to build up their self-esteem, needing to exercise a bit more of a say in relationships, some respect in relationships they were in, and also some stress management issues handling that thing of multiple roles in their lives without going mad or breaking down. A lot of them were socially isolated and didn't really have anybody or other people in their lives to talk to about these sorts of issues. So it seemed to me that they might actually get more out of talking about these sorts of things with each other in a group, in hopefully what would be a mutually supportive group, than just coming to see me week after week, being alone in a counselling room. That can tend to be a bit pathologising.

The women who make up the Breast Cancer Therapy Group—
Jean, Jeanne, Jeanette, Susanne, Lesley, Mary, Lois and Gail—warmly
responded to my request and set aside time after their regular weekly
meeting for us to talk. We met around the table in one of the conference rooms in the large public hospital where their meetings are held.
It was a gathering marked by laughter as well as sadness, openness,
thoughtfulness and a sense of cameraderie.

People come together with (a common problem) and of course we
have metastatic breast cancer ... so then we understand each
other through all our ups and downs. It has a sense of making
whatever our problems are manageable. To a certain degree, breast
cancer for us is able to be coped with and the terrible traumatic
problems we had before we came to the group [which] we were
handling on our own, [are diminished] because others are there
and you're not just on your own.

They believe that their group is the best means for achieving this
understanding and for helping to make their problems easier to cope
with. They comment:

the main link we have is our breast cancer and all the stuff that
happens to us—issues like hair loss, body image, wellness ...
This group is very confronting—you know all the problems of
everyone and you're suddenly more confronted with your own
situation; you realise you're mortal and it's life-threatening ...
We've talked quite openly about death and dying. Some girls
who've been in our group have died. J talked quite openly about
dying right up until she died ... and she made us feel better
about it because everyone's got to die sooner or later. She put a
different slant on it ... she showed us how to have a good death
... she was young—she was inspirational ...

Getting started

These brief introductions and accounts of their group work and participation give us a hint of the depth of knowledge and experience each person holds. For the most part, their purposes in forming or joining a group have arisen from personal experience and reflection, reinforced by their continued participation in the work of the group. Heather, for example, exemplifies the reflective practitioner, mining her knowledge base for different and more meaningful ways to meet the needs of her service users. Maria realised that there was an absence of information pertaining to the fertility issues which she, and others like her, confronted. For the women in the Breast Cancer Therapy Group, their rationale and purposes in joining and staying in the group were strengthened by their experience in the group. The group 'gives people the courage to live with [breast cancer] . . . with a positive attitude you feel much better so you're not worrying about it all the time . . . you learn to enjoy life and I think we do—we don't put anything off'.

It can also be useful to check prior research in order to discover what evidence there is or what others can tell us about whether a group might work well in achieving particular purposes. Robyn, for example, reviewed the relevant literature on step-parenting and discovered that two different group programs already existed. As a consequence, she developed her group as an amalgam of these two, drawing together both an educational and a therapeutic focus. The Breast Cancer Therapy Group is itself part of ongoing research studying the impact of supportive–expressive group therapy for women with recurrent breast cancer (Spiegel and Spira 1991; see also Posluszny et al. 1998).

Purpose

What is particularly striking in hearing how these group leaders and participants have described the purpose their group is set up to meet is the range of purposes identified. These purposes include insight

(Bernard and Lou), learning (Robyn), support (Cynthia, Heather, Breast Cancer Therapy Group), social action (Helen, Bob, Maria), performance and personal development (Bridget), research (Janet) and behaviour change (Chris). Some groups, such as Bob's, Maria's and Heather's, identify several connected purposes and we noted at the outset how Helen's group incorporated at least eight purposes.

The purposes which groups can serve are numerous (see Forsyth 1999, p. 102). Indeed, it is difficult to identify purposes which cannot be achieved by working collectively. However, the choice to form a group centres on determining an appropriate and realistic purpose. Determining the 'right' purpose at the outset significantly affects what kind of a group eventuates. In practice settings, we often decide (perhaps intuitively) that a group is the best way to go about something. When pressed, we can struggle to clearly articulate the specific purpose(s) we have in mind. However, to be able to do this is very important. As Kurland and Salmon (1998) argue, in situations where purposes are vague or non-existent, a group may struggle to survive. A clearly focused purpose helps to keep us on track, which may be an indispensable support when we are in the thick of a dynamic and turbulent group.

Changing purposes

While groups may be formed to achieve a specific purpose or several purposes, these purposes may also change over time as the group develops and evolves and as the social context in which it is embedded changes. Spiegel and Spira (1991, p. 47) identify that one of the purposes informing their expressive–supportive group therapy for women with recurrent breast cancer was to assist participants to move from passive acceptance of the initial group purpose to an active determination of the group's purpose and a critical evaluation of what was personally relevant to them from the combined input of others in the group.

Maria's self-help group moved from being a social group meeting the needs of families sharing similar issues around fertility to becoming an advocacy group which has established itself as a legitimate interest group consulted by policy-making bodies: 'We wouldn't have got there unless we'd organised—there's no way. Who would listen to one person?'

Robyn's step-parenting group, with its educational and skill-based program, has seen various cohorts of participants develop a further purpose for themselves—that of ongoing social support. To this end, a number of those who have been through the program continue to meet in an informal social support network (see also Scott et al. 2001).

However, a change in a group's purpose may not always be helpful, especially if the majority of participants do not wish to pursue a different purpose. When Maria's group made the transition from a social group to an advocacy and social action group, a number of participants left the group. Other groups, such as Helen's social action group, conclude once they have achieved the group's purpose, perhaps because the momentum had slackened or the participants are satisfied with their achievements. She comments:

> We were really clear that the issue was what the group was for. There was a move towards the end to shift into a lobby group for consumers . . . but that didn't take, so we folded.

Conflicting purposes

Where the potential exists for conflict in the interpretation or under-standing of a group's purpose, the group worker needs to ensure that, as far as possible, everyone is clear about the purpose at the outset— or at the very least, is able to work toward achieving some commonality of purpose as the group unfolds. As Janet described in relation to her focus groups, participants may have very different pur-poses from those of the leader. In some situations—particularly where the interests of leaders and potential participants are distant from or in opposition to one another—the possibility that conflict will occur is increased, and may mean that a group should not be established. However, it is also possible that all parties may decide to work together with the express purpose of finding common ground and shared goals which can be achieved collectively.

Chris, in his group for men who are violent, ensures that the men—many of whom are referred as part of a court order to attend the group—meet with him prior to entering the group. He notes: 'Nobody wants to come through that door to see me.' However, his purpose in meeting with them is to begin the process of building rapport: 'Giving them some sense there's an opportunity here for them . . . to deal with their own stuff. [It is also an opportunity] for them to suss me out.'

Agreeing On purpose

To decide to form a group, rather than work on an issue or task independently, suggests that, at some level, we believe that the purpose we have in mind will be achieved best by the collective involvement of a number of people. When we articulate the purpose, we are specifying the kind of group we want to either form or join. The design or form the group is to take derives from the purpose. Purpose determines the kinds of people who might be selected or wish to join it, the kind of leadership it will have and the type of group it will be (Douglas 2000; Magen 1995).

Achieving agreement on the group's purpose is essential if the members are to work successfully together. For example, there may be difficulties in setting up a group for residents in an institutional or custodial setting. The purposes behind decisions (usually initiated by staff) to develop a group may be in conflict with those held by the potential participants. Custodial settings are generally designed as mechanisms of social control and behaviour change, while residential institutions such as aged persons' facilities and nursing homes often accommodate people who are there against their wishes. To establish a group in such settings will require careful assessment as to ways in which a common purpose can be developed in light of likely conflicting interests of leaders and participants.

Of course, forming a group may not always be the right way to address a problem or issue, depending on the nature of the issue and the context. The worker needs to constantly ask: is group work indicated here? Is a group the correct or best way to achieve the outcomes envisaged? Some factors which may indicate that a group will not be successful refer to:

- the extent to which the auspicing agency welcomes and supports such an initiative. Where this is lacking, it is possible that a group will struggle and may be overtly or covertly undermined;
- the availability of resources to maintain a group. These include time, space and funds, as well as an appraisal of the skills which the group worker has, their level of competence and the extent of their experience;
- the nature of the problems, issues and resources which potential group participants have. For example, if members have an intellectual disability or severe hearing loss, what kinds of purposes are achievable?

Groups work best when the question 'Why would you do it on your own?' has become redundant—that is, when the group has a clear purpose justifying and framing its existence. Or, as Bridget reflects in relation to the Women's Circus:

> being part of a community, it's a lot of fun, sense of belonging, being physical, being fitter, different ways of using my body; it does heaps for my mental health . . . the common purpose of the group is to be a group.

Maria is similarly affirming:

> It's just fantastic—you're not the only one in the world who feels this way and that's incredible—it empowers people to know that somebody else [has] these negative feelings you had . . . because then they don't become the monsters you have to keep secret and you can't talk to your husband about.

Groups can return again and again and re-work the purpose, acknowledging individual differences and altered circumstances whilst trying to find common ground to continue on together—or, as we saw with Helen's group, to terminate. Whether the group's purpose remains constant from the beginning or whether it is something negotiated and renegotiated over the life of the group depends on the kind of group it is.

Summary

In this chapter, we have been introduced to the group leaders, workers and participants with whom I spoke when preparing this book and whose comments illustrate many of the points made throughout. Here their thoughts on the centrality of groups having clearly articulated purposes are drawn upon and some of the issues which need to be considered in relation to group purpose are described. Knowing a group's purpose also tells us something about the theoretical orientation and perspective of the leader or members, and this is the subject of the next chapter.

3

THEORETICAL BASIS OF
GROUP WORK:
'It's more like growing plants than
running a machine'

In the previous chapter, we discussed the importance of identifying and developing a purpose for a group. It was argued that purpose acts as a central core, justifying and holding the group together.

The identification of purpose also gives us a clue as to the theoretical perspective underpinning the decision to establish the group. This perspective comprises one's ideas, beliefs, values and assumptions about the nature of social reality. People have theories about why things are as they are, and within these theories are ideas about how change—and change into what—can be achieved or, conversely, what ought not to be changed. The very idea of using a group rather than some other strategy suggests we hold some kind of theory about where groups fit into our understanding of the social world. There can be no 'theoryless' group work practice. Sometimes the theoretical perspective is one of the primary reasons for the existence of the group. Bob comments in regard to his group Men Against Sexual Assault:

It has an explicit pro-feminist focus and brings this theoretical focus into the group . . . the pro-feminist stuff shapes the way we talk to each other about our experiences as men . . . (see also Pease and Camilleri 2001, pp. 6–7).

Sometimes a theoretical perspective may not be explicit or only vaguely specified, but it is always present. Theories are reflected in the knowledge bases which group leaders and participants draw upon and the language they use to explain them. They are exemplified in the choices that are made about forming a group, about joining a group, about the purposes to be pursued and about the means used to achieve them. Theory provides a window into a world view.

For example, Cynthia, in her group for children whose mothers are enduring cancer treatments or palliative care, expressed her theoretical perspective as being 'all based on meaning beyond the presence of mother'. The language she uses and the program she has developed suggest an affinity with humanistic and existential perspectives. Cynthia notes:

The tasks mother does for them are replaceable but the relationship is not. Therefore the relationship needs to be commemorated . . . creating memories—that's the gift.

Theories for group work

There are many theories for conceptualising what groups are and for working with them. Perhaps because of their abundance, the field sometimes appears confused. This apparent theoretical over-supply can inhibit rather than assist our use of them in practice. A further complication in distinguishing theoretical perspectives arises from the fact that different types of groups—for example, psychotherapy and psychoeducational groups—can (and often do) proceed from similar theoretical bases.

Defining groups

We might begin trying to sort through this theoretical 'plenty' by attempting to define what a group is. Again, there are a great number of definitions. Forsyth (1999, p. 6), for example, details eight in what he refers to as 'a sampling of definitions'.

To give a flavour of the differences among definitions which suggest quite distinctive world views, I have noted four:

A group is two or more persons who are interacting with each other in such a manner that each person influences and is influenced by each other person. (Shaw 1981, p. 454)

A group is a social system involving regular interaction among members and a common group identity. This means that groups have a sense of 'weness' that enables members to identify themselves as belonging to a distinct entity. (Johnson 1995, p. 1125)

The ability to gather up, name, give a sense to and transform states of mind and feelings is an essential characteristic of the psychoanalytic group. (Neri 2000, p. 8)

My own preferred definition of a group would identify it as:

a bounded social experience which includes:

- an objective element—it exists in time and space and is usually visible and tangible;
- a subjective element, which is felt, created and co-constructed in the minds, bodies and intellects of participants.

Definitions offer potential meanings at best, but they do point us towards grasping various theoretical perspectives which are embedded—although rarely articulated—values, beliefs and assumptions. For example, Johnson's definition (above) suggests an adherence to systems theory, Shaw's to learning theory, Neri's to psychoanalytic theory, and my own to a social constructionist perspective, all of which we will consider later in the chapter.

One of the questions I discussed in several recent conversations with people who lead or participate in groups was how they would define a group. Again, their responses reflected the possible range of definitions:

> It's a bit like another family that you go into . . . in a supportive sense . . . (Bernard)

> It's hard to define who you are . . . we wanted a space where there were no outsiders and we couldn't be judged . . . we wanted a safe place . . . (Maria)

> A group's an organic thing . . . it's far more like growing plants than running a machine . . . (Helen)

> Very much a living thing . . . (Lou)

Interestingly, from the 'within' group perspective, very different ways of defining what a group is are apparent. What stands out is the sense of the group as an experience or a process rather than an object. Participants in my conversations used metaphors to capture the essence of this experience. To them, the group experience is likened to a family, a refuge, growing plants, a living organism. It seems closer to the 'lived experience' of group leading and participating to use language which belongs more to the realm of the poetic and the felt rather than to the lexicon of classification and abstraction (see Croker 1977). This alerts us to the many levels at which group process operates, and the dynamic and moving nature of the process.

Generally, we might agree that the role of theory is to achieve a level of abstraction which excludes, as far as possible, ambiguity. The poetic, on the other hand, thrives on ambiguity and suggestion. Artistic representations in poetry, art and sculpture do not come with directives for action; rather, their imperative is interpretation. Very importantly, for theory to have a bearing on practice, it must take into account the 'lived experience' of group leaders and participants—their actual experience of the phenomenon of the group. This is what we all (facilitators, leaders, participants) work with. But to begin to construct this linkage we need to look more closely at theory and what we want theory to 'do' for us.

What do we want theory to do for us?

One way of answering this question is to consider that there are different aspects of our work or different moments in our practice where theoretical knowledge is helpful. At an abstract level of generality, theory may:

- provide a way of thinking about what we do or want to do;
- assist our understanding about what is taking place in the group;
- give coherence to the complexity we encounter;
- locate what is being observed within some framework of meaning;
- provide us with the conceptual means to go beyond what is self-evident.

In order to *inform our actions in the group and in the 'wider' context* in which it is situated, theory may:

- indicate possible causes for what we observe or do;
- indicate possible relationships amongst phenomena we observe or things we do;
- identify the 'grammar' of the action we observe—those unnamed 'rules' governing what is said or done;

- indicate for us what is important to note, observe, understand amongst the plethora of phenomena and experiences occurring in the group;
- indicate those forces or factors which influence how we act even if we are not aware of them—for example, unconscious elements, factors outside awareness, factors in the 'wider' economic and political world which are impacting upon us whether or not we are aware of them;
- ensure that we are accountable for what we do, and that we can offer a justification for the 'reasonableness' of our actions.

As a way of *mediating between 'lived experience' of practice or participation and the more abstract level of generality*, theory may:

- provide guidelines on how to act;
- provide a rationale for acting in a particular way;
- provide a language for talking about what we do and what we understand with others who speak the same language;
- provide information upon which to reflect and critically appraise or evaluate what is going on and our actions in relation to this;
- connect with our 'lived experience' as workers and as participants;
- give us choices about how to act and what to do.

There are, of course, other ways in which theory might be useful to us, and some of those noted here may not be in accord with everyone's position. Where we place our priority depends on our knowledge, values, beliefs, experiences and the context in which we are working.

The thumb-nail sketches of various theoretical positions outlined in the next section may be usefully critiqued by 'interrogating' them in relation to the purposes we believe theoretical knowledge should serve. To what extent do these theoretical perspectives 'work' for us? How well do they accord with our own values and beliefs about what groups are for, about how we want to work with them, about where group work practice fits our conceptualisations of social relationships?

five theoretical vantage points

This section of the chapter proposes a guide through this theoretical abundance by suggesting that there are at least five vantage points from which to read the available theory. These five perspectives were selected because they seem to capture the most prevalent perspectives evident in contemporary group work practice. (More detailed accounts of the range of theories useful in group work can be found in Hanson et al. 1980; Toseland and Rivas 1998; and Corey 2000, as well as many other texts.)

The difficulty with approaching the literature in this way is that, by design, it pigeonholes ideas and theories to the exclusion of other positions and vantage points which they might also fit. The clarity which is obtained here is (hopefully to only a small extent) at the expense of the perspective described. The criticism may be reasonably made that justice is not always fully done. However, the rationale for the selection and categorisation of perspectives in this way is that it identifies what is argued to be the central concern or preoccupation of that perspective. These are 'ideal types' rather than fully fledged accounts. This always goes with a recognition that there may also be other concerns and preoccupations which get marginalised in the desire for some clarity and distinction amongst competing views. It does not mean that they are mutually exclusive and many practitioners, quite reasonably, borrow and mix and match amongst available theoretical formulations, describing their approach as 'eclectic'. What each vantage point offers is a way of seeing the group which brings with it imperatives or guidelines for how one defines what a group is and how group leaders and participants work in and with a group. So, in describing each of these vantage points, an example of each perspective is included as it (or elements of it) has been used in practice.

The five vantage points from which group work theories will be surveyed are:

- the group as a power base;
- the group as a system;
- the group as a container of individuals;
- the group as container of properties;
- the group as a site of meaning construction.

The group as a power base

The theoretical perspectives which take the concept of the group as a power base originate in Marxist political philosophy and sociology. Such theories begin from the premise that problems which individuals experience are social and structural rather than personal. Thus the focus of the group is upon taking political action which leads to social change rather than making attempts to change individual behaviours (Vinik and Levin 1991; Weeks 1994, Ch. 3; Butler and Wintram 1995; DeChant 1996; Benjamin et al. 1997). An analysis of power structures which operate in capitalist societies demonstrates that certain segments of the population are discriminated against, oppressed and marginalised both because of, and in order to reinforce, their unequal access to power and resources. Women, disabled people, poor people, people of colour and those who belong to minority ethnic or racial groups are frequently rendered less powerful, ignored, stigmatised and excluded from achieving influence in the wider society. The particular problems or issues they face in individual relationships may better be understood as the product of social and power relationships prevailing in capitalist societies rather than individual pathology (Burkhardt 1982; Fook 1993; Mullaly 1993; Ife 1997; Pease and Fook 1999).

Self-help groups, advocacy groups and social action groups may emerge as a response to these structural conditions and, as such, embody sites of resistance to the status quo. According to Sullivan (1984, p. 139): 'Resistance can be . . . the beginning of an authentic project which is indicative of a developing sense of agency. Resistance becomes an agent process when it fosters the development of community and solidarity.'

These groups take as their focus the development of collective action. This might include using the group process of sharing perspectives as a means of consciousness-raising. Consciousness-raising facilitates the development of insight into the nature of their circumstances and the structural factors which have brought them about. Participants may then decide to take action to change these circumstances. A key theoretical component is the concept of *praxis*—the process whereby the theoretical understanding achieved by the group is implemented in the action taken. Reflection on that action may result in theoretical change, a change in action, and so on. The group then becomes the site where perspectives, actions and outcomes are shared and the dialectical process which ensues has the potential to emancipate and empower. Participation in the group may enable members to increase both their social equality and the control they may exert over their lives.

Example

Mullender and Ward (1991) describe their approach to group work as the 'self-directed approach'. Positioning themselves within a critical theory perspective, they advocate group work which can:

> bridge the gap between group members as individuals and wider social institutions: that is, between private troubles and public issues . . . In practice, this means emphasising the members' own definitions of their situation, facilitating their understanding and working uncompromisingly with issues as they define them (1991, p. 126).

Drawing on their practice experience with a range of client groups, they articulate six practice principles derived from their value position and commitment to using group work to bring about social change and personal betterment and empowerment. These principles (paraphrased) are:

1 a recognition of the skills, understanding and ability of the people with whom they work;
2 a rights perspective which advocates the rights of service users to decide whether or not to participate in self-directed work, and the right to define issues and act on them;
3 the centrality of practice reflecting the contribution of structural factors (oppression, social policy, the economy, the environment) to service users' problems;
4 a commitment to the belief that power can be acquired through collective action;
5 all work must challenge oppression in whatever form it exists;
6 methods of work must reflect non-elitist principles. The group worker facilitates the process of decision-making and the responsibility for and control of outcomes.

From these practice principles flows a three-stage model:

Stage one: Taking stock: From a process reflective of the workers' value position, people 'who share a particular structural problem [are invited] to choose to join the group' (1991, p. 131).

Stage two: Taking action: The group moves to explore the questions: *What* problem is to be addressed? *Why* is it a problem? *How* is it to be tackled? Group members themselves take those actions decided upon.

Stage three: Taking over: The group reviews the connections between *What? Why? How?*

• New issues may need to be tackled—*Reformulating 'What?'*

- The group perceives the links between the different issues—*Reformulating 'Why?'*
- The group decides what actions to take next—*Reformulating 'How?'*

Criticisms of group work practice drawing on structural accounts of social and political relations refer to the absence of focus on individual problems, and a tendency to ignore the 'inner workings' of groups. One of the limitations of this approach might be that it fails to adequately encompass individuals' thoughts, feelings and explanations about how they see themselves and how they manage their individual 'problems in living'. This suggests that, in some situations—for example, where participants are confronting life-threatening illness—this theoretical approach might not be the primary perspective underlying the group's formation. However, it might at other times be apparent if participants adopted an advocacy or patient rights focus.

The group as a system

Systems theory, which originated in the fields of biology and engineering, is perhaps the most widely used and broadly applied theory of group functioning (Toseland and Rivas 1998, pp. 56–59). Most group workers include elements of the central concepts of systems theory in conceptualising their practice.

Systems theory focuses primarily on the group as an entity, as a system of interacting elements. As such, it relies on mechanical and natural science metaphors, depicting the group as being in constant interaction with another system—its environment. The group works to maintain its equilibrium despite the constant and changing demands exerted on it by the external system. To do so, according to Toseland and Rivas (1998), groups must take action in four ways. Groups need to be integrated so that members' close connectedness with one another ensures that a boundary is maintained. This boundary can be penetrated, however, as the group will need to adapt and change, grow and shrink in order to cope with environmental demands. To keep the sense of group identity and agreed-upon procedures in place, the group's basic purpose needs to be clearly defined and sustained. This is what is meant by pattern maintenance. The fourth action the group takes—goal attainment—describes the group as a system with a purpose which must be accomplished. The tasks and the processes required to attain the group's goal are kept clearly to the forefront of the group's activities.

Systems theory suggests that members are frequently subject to powerful forces exerted by the group itself. The group seeks harmony and balance in the face of the conflict inherent in its struggle to maintain equilibrium in relation to the impingement of other external systems. In the process, however, the group is kept in a constant state of becoming and developing which may be problematic for its quest to continue existing.

Many theories of groups are derived from systems theory: social network intervention (Scott 1988; Scott et al. 2001); mutual aid (Shulman 1999); and the group as a resource system (Douglas 1993, 2000). This is partly because systems theory has been such a powerful and pervasive theory in understanding social life.

Example

An example of systems theory as applied to social group work is provided by Shulman's depiction of the group as a mutual aid system (1999).

Shulman begins with his notion of the group as a 'microsociety' in which members have the potential to help one another through their interaction around the common problems that they bring to the group. While members need each other, there are obstacles to mutual aid taking place, such as the possibility that the group will exert coercion rather than be conducive to providing a safe

---

environment where trust, bonding and cohesion can prevail. In Shulman's view, it is the group worker's task to 'help the group members create the conditions in which mutual aid can take place' (1999, p. 303).

Shulman outlines ten ways in which group members can help each other: through the sharing of data; the dialectical process; discussing a taboo area; the 'all-in-the-same-boat' phenomenon; developing a universal perspective; mutual support; mutual demand; individual problem-solving; rehearsal; and the 'strength-in-numbers' phenomenon.

Through these ten processes, mutual aid is offered and taken. However, the group leader must work to enable members to identify what they have in common with others so that they can learn both to seek assistance and to offer it. This is one way the members can benefit and develop skills which will be of use in the wider social context of their lives outside the group.

As the group is conceptualised as a complex system, it must learn to deal with several developmental tasks if it is to survive and be productive. Shulman (1999, p. 313) notes that: 'As soon as more than one client is involved a new organism is created . . . The group is more than the sum of its parts . . . the new organism needs to to develop rules and procedures that will allow it to function effectively.' The group leader must assist the group to deal with change in ways that are adaptive and growth-enhancing—in brief, to help the group become a mutual aid system. As such, the group leader's role is to mediate between the individual and the group as a whole. (See also Kelly 1999; Douglas 2000; Manor 2000.)

A critique of systems theory usually begins with argument over the applicability to the social world of metaphors drawn from the natural and physical sciences. Social life may be seen as having very little to do with the characteristics of a machine or a rainforest.

In addition, systems theory is sometimes seen as limited in its ability to account for conflict and change as a goal and a strategy. This may mean that a social action or advocacy group would find systems theory's perspective in opposition to their theorisation of power and its impetus for action.

The group as a container of individuals

The theoretical perspectives which focus primarily on the individuals who comprise the group are clearly the obverse of systems theory, which takes the group as an entity as its object. Here, the emphasis is on group members who bring individual motivations, personalities, mental processes and behaviours to the group, and it is these elements in interaction which create and characterise collective group processes. Two key examples of theories derived from individual psychology and applied to the group are psychoanalytic theory and learning theory. They are frequently in evidence in psychotherapy and counselling groups, and in psychoeducational groups.

The theoretical perspectives which begin with individuals are derived from psychological theories of personality, human develop-ment and psychopathology. They are then used and adapted to explain collective group processes. Where systems theory recognises the group itself as a powerful force acting to affect individual behaviour, here individual differences and similarities are recognised as powerfully affecting the group. However, in focusing on the group as comprising individuals, it is not always clear whether the improvement hoped for in individuals' lives is to occur through working with them individu-ally in the group, or through working with the group as a whole in order to change individuals (Anthony 1971). This lack of clarity can generate confusion, not only in the literature but also in practice, as to whether or not and in what ways the individual should be the target of the leader's interventions. Other criticisms of this perspective point to the absence of an adequate understanding of the context within which individuals and groups are situated. Groups described and analysed from this perspective appear to locate the group and the individuals in an 'empty world'. The language of pathology, which characterises psychoanalytic theory and the sense that individuals can be coerced and trained through rewards and punishments implicit in learning theory, may sit uncomfortably with those who consider such language to be oppressive and stigmatising, or as proposing the trans-cultural adoption of normative standards of behaviour.

Psychoanalytic theory (Anthony 1971; Toseland and Rivas 1998; Corey 2000, pp. 145–84) proceeds from an understanding of the family as the individual's first experience of a group. The original family, which can also be thought of as a group, was the site for the experience of conflict as the individual negotiated psychosexual stages of development and maturation. In the group, these early family experiences are re-enacted. The concepts of *transference* and *counter-transference* (which refer to the dynamic impact, often unconscious, which is seen as emerging between individuals, and between individuals and the leader) are important in understanding the ways in which individuals re-encounter unresolved conflicts and are assisted in linking these struggles to their current behaviour. The purpose of the group is for individuals, through their engagement with others, to gain insight into the causes and manifestations of these unresolved conflicts. Through the group process, they strengthen their inter-personal skills and adaptive capacities.

Groups drawing on psychoanalytic theory tend to be relatively unstructured. Group members bring their own agendas and are encouraged to speak as freely as possible about any issues or concerns they have. The group may meet more frequently than once a week. They are open groups where membership fluctuates. It is not unusual for members to attend for long periods, perhaps several years. The group leader takes a somewhat non-interactive and distant stance which facilitates participants' projections and fantasies. These often unconsciously derived projections are evident in transference and counter-transference reactions. The group leader's role is to offer interpretations which focus on these unconscious productions, enabling members' anxieties and distortions to become visible and, in this way, assist the participant to gain insight into him/herself.

Learning theory also takes individuals in the group as its focus. With considerable debt to cognitive behavioural psychology, learning theory emphasises that individuals can learn to think and act differently if they want to change problematic behaviour or reframe situations differently. In the group, rewards and punishments for 'good' and 'bad' behaviour are communicated by reinforcement offered in various forms—for example, attention from the leader, supportive comments from other members when 'positive' learning or acting takes place. Of course, 'good' and 'bad' behaviour reflect normative assumptions about what is acceptable or desirable. Groups deriving from this theoretical perspective tend to emphasise clear structure and planning, so goals will be specified, a contract may be drawn up to ensure members actively use the group to attain these goals, desired outcomes are specified in ways that make them measurable, and the group's progress will be evaluated (Coyne 1999; see also Peled and Davis 1995).

Example: A psychoeducational group for women in substance abuse treatment

Plasse (2000) presents an account of the Parenting in Recovery Program (PIR) which she describes as a psychoeducational group with the dual agenda of educating and fostering self-understanding through the dynamics of the group.

This psychoeducational group has been designed to assist participants who have long-standing substance abuse problems to make the transition from addiction to recovery but with the recognition that, if they are to function well as parents, they require education. Group members may attend the group voluntarily or as a result of a court order.

As participants join the group because of extreme difficulties in their lives, the importance of maintaining their involvement and ensuring that the program addresses the problematic issues in their lives is central. The program devised is planned to include elements which 'engage and sustain member participation and lead to program completion by group members' (2000, p. 48).

PIR has a fifteeen-session program. Topics focus on parental self-awareness, attachment theory, child development, positive discipline and the acquisition of communication skills. It is a highly structured curriculum which concludes with the awarding of a certificate of completion. Group members are required to attend a minimum of thirteen sessions which are held on a weekly or twice-weekly basis. Participants complete fourteen journal assignments and each session commences with participants reading their journal entries to the group. Group leaders read and provide feedback on the journal work. 'Respect and esteem building rather than critical confrontation characterise the values of the program and the style of leadership' (2000, p. 36).

The group as container of properties

Various theoretical perspectives focus on groups as comprising properties which are common to all of them. Conceptualising groups in this way proposes that these properties can be abstracted from individual or particular groups and analysed in their own right. Common properties, such as the prevalence of communication and interaction, the centrality of cohesion (the attractiveness of groups to its members) and the emergence of group culture (those shared perspectives and ways of understanding that come to characterise the unique 'flavour' of a group) can be identified. As these properties are considered common to all groups, they allow for comparative studies to be undertaken, suggesting the factors which enhance or inhibit positive outcomes for group functioning. Other group properties refer to the tendency of group members to adopt norms and roles within the group and take on behaviours which reflect individual status within the group, such as the scapegoat, the leader, the deviant member, and so on (Forsyth 1998, pp. 119–44). These are seen as exerting a powerful influence on participants and on the way the entire group functions.

The interplay of group dynamics may change in character and intensity at various moments over the life of the group. This has led various group theorists to propose that all groups can be understood as evolving through various stages or phases. These phases have been depicted as linear and sequential or as cyclical (Berman-Rossi 1992; Brower 1996). However, it is their perceived universality that has enabled them to be studied as distinct, yet shared, properties of all groups.

Example

Manor (2000), while locating his approach within systems theory, proposes a framework for working with 'timelimited interpersonal groups that include increasing awareness of communication in the group'. This he terms 'an inclusive stance' (2000, p. 15). He argues that, although there are differences in groups, 'groups do show sufficient similarities so that we may compare and contrast one with all others: groups are also similar to one another' (2000, p. 16).

Manor takes the communication property shared by all groups as the central and connecting element in his framework. He considers that communication involves a paradox: in order to understand how group members influence one another (an important tenet of systems theory), group workers need to examine how members interact—but in order to understand that interaction, group workers need to distinguish the individuals who comprise the group.

By analysing the communication needs of all groups, Manor presents what he terms 'an inclusive blueprint of group stages'

(2000, p. 21). This blueprint is intended to assist group workers choose what to do and how to lead by understanding the dynamics of groups as they are presented at different stages in the group's evolution. The eight stages Manor identifies are derived from conceptualising group work as 'evolving within a three-cornered world'—contents, structure and process (2000, p. 28).

Criticisms of this perspective refer to the extent to which diverse groups do indeed share common properties which can be abstracted and studied in their own right and outside of any context. For example, to assume that all groups develop in phases or stages which can be identified and named may detract from seeing the uniqueness and creativity of individual groups. Such stages and phases may not be able to be generalised—for example, where factors such as gender, race or class are concerned. However, as we shall discuss later in this book, the relationship between time, the duration of the group and change are of considerable significance in understanding the ways in which groups work.

When groups are studied as entities characterised by shared properties, the question of what makes groups 'work' in terms of achieving the group's purpose and the participants' goals can be posed. Yalom's work (1975), used in the following illustration, arises from this question.

Example

Yalom (1975), with a commitment to psychoanalytic theory, focuses upon understanding the practice of group psychotherapy by identifying the change mechanisms shared across the range of psycho-therapeutic group work approaches, including psychoanalytic therapy, family therapy, Gestalt therapy, and many more. He referred to these change mechanisms as 'curative factors' (1975, p. xi). Yalom argues that: 'Therapy groups which appear totally different in form may rely on identical mechanisms of change.' The eleven curative factors he identifies (1975, pp. 3–4) are well known:

- instillation of hope;
- universality;
- imparting of information;
- altruism;
- corrective recapitulation of the primary family group;
- development of socialising techniques;
- imitative behaviour;
- interpersonal learning;
- group cohesiveness;
- catharsis;
- existential factors.

While not disregarding the fact that group goals may differ in relation to the leader's adherence to a particular therapeutic canon and the importance of the composition of the group, Yalom considers these curative factors to be the primary agents of change. Recognising, understanding and developing one's practice to maximise the impact of these curative factors is, from Yalom's perspective, vital to advancing theory and technique on group psychotherapy.

The group as site of meaning construction

When I embarked on preliminary research for this book, I began by initiating a number of conversations with people who lead, facilitate or participate in groups. My aim, following a loosely structured set of questions, was to engage with them in discussion about what being in a group meant to them from their different perspectives. This proved a rich and fascinating experience and their comments have provided an interesting and colourful association to various points made throughout the text. Such an approach to the development of the book signals my own perspective and interest in groups as sites of meaning construction. Interestingly, this perspective is relatively underdeveloped in the extant group work literature. This is particularly striking when we consider that conversation and the telling of stories are central to the work of all groups.

Viewing groups as sites for the construction of meaning refers to constructionist and social constructionist theories and points towards postmodernist ideas. These theoretical perspectives and meta-theories (theories about theories) question empiricist and positivist arguments for certainty, for the utility of over-arching or grand theories about human nature and the nature of the social world. Constructionism is sourced in Kantian philosophy and proposes that people create their own realities through our subjective interpretations of their observations and experiences. Social constructionism derives from social psychology, which argues that social knowledge is relative to each social and linguistic group of knowers (Crotty 1998, pp. 42–57). Our ways of knowing and understanding are constrained and enhanced by the social, political and historical context in which we participate (Dean 1993; Laird 1995). Thus human knowledge is recognised as subjective and requiring interpretation. Social constructionism emphasises that this act of interpretation takes place intersubjectively—that is, between people. Meanings are negotiated in interaction with others. Within the 'wider' social context, discourses provide 'the reservoirs of meaning and language from which individuals and families fashion their stories. Knowing then is narrative.' (Laird 1995, p. 155) Discourse thus includes both theory and practice—what we think as well as what we do.

Postmodernism takes this awareness of the socially constructed nature of existence further. It proposes new ways of understanding the self; no longer is it seen as an autonomous, consistent and necessarily coherent entity but rather as fragmentary, decentred and always in process. According to Parton and Marshall (1998, p. 244), language is central to the sense of self (or multiple selves), to thought and to subjectivity: 'Language is seen as mediating and constituting all that is "known" . . . We cannot transcend the influence of interpretation and assume that reality is simply waiting to be discovered: it is constituted and constructed within language.' In relation to theories for group work, Parton and Marshall's (1998) work is helpful. They identify four central preoccupations of postmodernist practice:

Uncertainty is central. In relation to group work we would acknowledge that we cannot know in advance what the outcomes of interactions will be but we do know that whatever interpretations and meanings do emerge, they will be historically contingent and context bound. Their fluidity derives from the fluidity of language. The work of the group may thus comprise constructing meaning through dialogue from which may emerge a shared understanding of reality.

Deconstruction: this is a way of analysing texts, language and narrative so that none are taken as givens. Rather, in relation to the group, the group worker analyses language with reference to the social, historical and political context in which it occurs. Through this process the group experience may enable participants to externalise their problems and examine their influence on their life as evident in the language and discourse to which they refer.

Possibility: change is possible. By the process of deconstruction, reconstruction and listening, participants in groups may begin to redefine who they are and how they want to act.

Subjectivity: within postmodernist ways of thinking, the self is understood as being multifaceted and multivoiced, always in process. This means that one's subjectivity is constituted by contradiction, by fragmentation, by a sense of precariousness, fluidity and change depending upon the sociocultural, historical and interpersonal context in which one finds oneself. Thus, the group provides a particular setting in which one's subjectivity may be experienced and explored in the context of other subjects.

Postmodern group work thus proceeds from a recognition that the intersubjective context of the group can be a site for the construction and reconstruction of meaning. By talking and communicating, people may come to understand their experiences, to control and reframe them, and to take them further. The emphasis is placed on process and on participants as agents reauthoring their lives. As Parton and Marshall (1998, p. 248) point out in relation to social work practice—and this is particularly relevant to group work— 'solutions are found in the making, the telling and the talking'. Laird (1995, p. 160) makes a similar point: 'Therapy, for lack of a better term, should be in part a matter of deconstruction, of consciousness-raising, of learning how one's own stories have been constrained or demeaned or deprivileged in varying contexts of knowledge and power.' (See also McNamee and Gergen 1992; Gersie 1997; Davis and Jansen 1998; Arminen 1998.)

Postmodernism has been criticised for its own fluidity and over-inclusiveness, its rejection of 'grand theories', its lack of strategies for

---

Example

Dean (1998) proposes a narrative approach to groups. Her purpose is 'to create a multiplicity of options for action and understanding as individuals come to apprehend both the enduring aspects of their self accounts and those that are fluid and evolving' (1998, p. 36).

Dean uses a number of examples of a narrative approach to groups drawn from her practice. She embeds her practice firmly within a social constructionist and postmodern perspective:

Implicit in the concept of a narrative approach to work with groups is the overarching supposition that meaning develops between people through conversation . . . a story is told, there is a conversation about it, new meaning is introduced, and the story changes and takes on a different (sometimes expanded) meaning. In group settings the possibilities for change are enhanced by the numbers of people who can participate in the intersubjective expansion of meaning (1998, p. 27).

In the telling of stories, participants may enhance their capacity for self-reflection and critical analysis, perhaps extending the boundaries of what can normally be talked about. By doing this, challenges may be posed both to the participant and to other members about how a situation can be understood and problematised. The possibility for social action outside the group may thereby emerge.

Dean's narrative approach to groups includes a critique of the group leader's role as 'expert', as well as providing various strategies and analysis of group work practices in eliciting narratives, understanding their meaning from varying perspectives, and using narratives to bring about change and improved well-being for participants:

> At times, the new stories may simply offer different solutions to old problems; at other times, new or altered stories may bring more passion and vigour and a deeper set of meanings to a person's life (1998, p. 36).

action or change and the sense that 'anything goes' and nothing is to be particularly privileged or valued. However, already within such narrative approaches to group work as proposed by Dean (and others, see Gersie 1997), there is recognition that narratives and stories may be strategic and hold potential for action and change.

Towards a critical postmodern theory for group work

There is much overlap and interplay between all five perspectives discussed so far as well as the potential for rapprochement between perspectives that may seem, on the surface, to be in opposition or even contradictory. For example, group workers working from the perspective of the group as a power base emphasise the potential (and actuality) of collective work to achieve structural change. Where consciousness-raising is part of the group's activity, it is a process of enabling participants to reframe their personal stories within a socio-political context. In this way, their individual experiences of, for example, depression may be seen as a response to social structures which stigmatise, marginalise and disempower. This approach shares ground with the work in narrative groups where the major focus might be on discovering or constructing new or different meanings as stories are told.

These similarities between critical theory and postmodernism have important implications for understanding identity and subjectivity. Individuals talking to one another within the bounded social reality of the group are 'selves in relation'. In Ezzy's terms (1998, p. 239), drawing on the work of Maines (1993), we are 'self-narrating organisms'. In their talk, individuals tell stories drawing on past memories and future plans which change in meaning as a consequence of the interaction and exchanges in the group over time. During this process, the story-tellers provide a continuity to their narrative of lived experience which unites and amplifies the person's interpretation of their past, present and future. In the process of conversation in the group, individuals reflect on their self-identity as it is reinterpreted in the telling and as others react to it. This is close to the way in which Giddens (1991) refers to self-identity as the 'reflexive project of the self'.

However, these processes do not occur in a vacuum. Our understanding of social life informed by critical theory emphasises that one's sense of self is historically and socially grounded. As Ezzy states (1998, p. 250), 'narrative identities are sustained and transformed through the influence of social relationships as mediated by institutional structures . . . [it is a] political and power-laden process'. Steve Burkhardt (1982, p. 137) argues persuasively that how a group functions is itself a reflection of the impact of social factors dominant in a particular historical period. The nature of the group experience—

the process which characterises it—will differ according to the climate of the historical period. Different forms of group action will emerge where different socio-political factors prevail. The shared historical period of group leader and participants has brought them together in the group but often in unequal positions. Where a critical postmodern group work may illuminate this situation is that, within the group, the conversations, stories and reflections shared by both leaders and participants can include personal and social factors, retold and reflected upon in order to discover the meaning they construct about the psychological and material conditions affecting their lives.

The similarities between critical theory and postmodernism offer potential for understanding the ways in which language, narrative and discourse are implicit in the structuring of relations of power (Leonard 1997). To collectively engage in deconstructing these constructed meanings through a process of critical reflection places attention on the 'interactive aspects of situations (your own influence on the situation—interpretations, behaviour, hidden assumptions), and how this influence might have affected power relations or perpetuated existing structures and thinking' (Fook 1999, p. 203). Work in groups engages with the 'real life' experience of participants and in so doing may open up the possibilities for equally 'real' change.

Connecting theory to purpose

We concluded the previous chapter by promising to relate the discussion on the importance of group workers articulating their purpose to theory for group work. In this chapter we have viewed the theories which group work has drawn upon from five sometimes competing, sometimes sympathetic vantage points. It is evident from this that the decision about purpose is almost exclusively determined by the theoretical position from which it proceeded.

This means that, in identifying the purpose a group is to pursue, an issue is being problematised in a particular way. For example,

Heather's decision was to establish a group to work with the emotional and mental health issues with which women in her agency were presenting. The group's purpose was to focus on relating these personal struggles to structural factors referring to women's multiple roles, the stresses in their lives, their social isolation or their subordinate position in relationships. Thus Heather did not conceptualise the women's problems as being due to psychological pathology or mental illness. As a consequence, the group program combined psychoeducational principles (drawn from learning theory) and a feminist perspective (drawn from critical theory) which provided the analysis and understanding of their situations, and the impetus to work collectively.

Again, Chris's group for men who are violent has its theoretical base in Learning Theory, a belief that behaviour and attitude change is possible. The group is purposefully structured to use the participants' collective responses to challenge the way members construct their attitudes and behaviour.

Lou's positive ageing group combines psychoanalytic theory and concepts drawn from learning theory in a program working with large numbers of around 80 participants. The emphasis is placed on moving from didactic input to (at times) one-to-one work with the leader in the context of the large group, to small group discussion. The program does not explicitly refer to critical theoretical perspectives—for example, it does not include either a focus on the ways in which ageing is constructed in society, or one on the impact of structural factors on individual's lives—for instance, with regard to stigma and marginalisation, although at times these may be discussed with individuals.

As we noted at the outset, no practice can be 'theoryless': theory is always accessible if we analyse the assumptions, beliefs and values which underpin the decision to establish a group, the type of group established, the purpose it is to pursue, the structure and process it follows and the leadership characterising it. Although the five perspectives were presented in this chapter as separate, in practice group workers tend to rely on a range and mixture of theories. None is mutually exclusive. While the final result might be described as an 'eclectic' approach to group work, this is viable because of the overlap and interplay between perspectives that, from a surface reading only, may appear to be contradictory. Developments in critical postmodern theory for group work illustrate this. Importantly, however, 'good' practice can only become 'better' practice if we as group workers and group participants engage in reflection and critical analysis of what we do, why we do it and why sometimes it 'works' and sometimes it doesn't. Theory has a central role to play in this endeavour.

Summary

This chapter provided an introduction to the range of theories that contemporary group work practitioners draw on. A meta-analysis of these theories was offered, viewing the various theories from five vantage points which are distinguished by the particular metaphor which, arguably, underpins each perspective. Thus these theories suggest that the group may be understood as a power base, as a system, a container of individuals, a container of properties and a site of meaning construction. Recent developments in critical postmodern theory are discussed, as they might refer to a 'coming together' of different perspectives which may form a basis for future theoretical developments. The relationship between group purpose and theory was briefly examined, the argument being that how we analyse or problematise an issue as the basis for proposing group work as an intervention or action strategy is theory-based.

LEADING:
'A series of tasks anyone can do'

Introduction

This and the following two chapters will focus on the process of leading a group. While leadership and power are synonymous, the question of who is the leader and where their power comes from is not always obvious. In democratic and participatory groups, leadership and power are created through the reciprocity of relationships between members and (at least initially) the designated leader. At different times and for different reasons, all participants to the collective enterprise can assume leadership positions and undertake leadership acts. The power to influence and lead the group arises from a variety of contributions which participants and the designated leader bring to the group. These contributions are on the level of ideas, structural positioning, personal characteristics and skills or capabilities. This last source of power and influence will be discussed in Chapter 5 and its implications for practice are explored in Chapter 6.

Leading

The concept and the practice of leading are central to work with groups. The moment we talk about leadership, we are talking about the capacity to influence group participants and the development of the group itself. When we say we are influencing something, we are referring to the ability to make a difference in some way, to change things inside and outside the group—in other words, to exert power. This power can potentially be liberating as well as oppressive. But, as Douglas (2000, p. 55; see also Toseland and Rivas 1998, p. 91) notes, 'the exercise of this power must be justified . . . through the medium of its use information, knowledge, guidance and development can be created, [and] the power of the members enhanced in dealing with the group and their problems themselves'.

The use of the term 'leader' often sits uncomfortably with those who work in the human services. To some it seems to be a term suggestive of an authoritarian or coercive approach which disempowers group participants. Benjamin et al. (1997, p. 127; see also Mullender and Ward 1991), for example, prefer to speak of group facilitation; Mondros and Berman-Rossi (1991, p. 205) propose that community development groups do not have a leader. Rather, the organiser is an enabler, teacher and resource provider. However, Forsyth (1999, p. 342) comments: 'The term leader should be reserved for those who act in the best interests of a group with the consent of that group. Leadership is a form of power, but power *with* people rather than *over* people.' We are all only too aware that power may be used to effect change for the worse through coercion, sanctioning, punishing or denying group members access to privileges, power and resources. The history of the world attests to numerous such outcomes. Nevertheless, when work with groups is informed by humanistic and social justice values, it is democratic and participatory and holds the potential to be empowering.

The issue, then, is not so much whether the leader's role is a powerful one, but rather who has power and where this power comes from.

Who has power?

there is something about the group dynamic that is a powerful learning thing and part of it may well be that the other members of the group are not psychiatrists or psychotherapists. They are ordinary people who are struggling with the same sorts of issues and there is this sense of cooperation and helping each other that is quite a powerful dynamic . . . (Bernard)

Reciprocity and power

The forces that bring leaders and group members together in the first place are interesting to explore. From a psychoanalytic perspective, Bion asserted that group members come together in order to find a leader, someone who will meet their needs for dependency and security. Anthony (1971, p. 13) notes: 'The search for a leader . . . brings the group members together, and, once they find him [sic] they cannot do without him [sic].' Bion's view (quoted in Anthony 1971, p. 13) may seem unexpected, given that we more generally understand groups as being convened by someone, usually the leader, and comprising participants recruited or invited to join by the leader. However, both points of view can be accommodated through the notion of reciprocity and the recognition that power in the group is relational.

The group comprises a number of individuals who, in their interaction, create the group. Each of the sources of power could equally well be contributed by each participant—and at different times in the life of the group this is indeed what happens. As Tindale et al. (1998, p. 4) point out: 'Different tasks require different leaders, and roles shift over time . . . depending upon the interests of the members and the skills they bring to the group.' Groups are essentially mutual enterprises in which the capacity for reciprocity in roles and relationships is a primary force in determining the effectiveness of the group in fulfilling both individual and mutually agreed purposes. In this respect, leadership is fundamentally derived from the interaction of the group

(Toseland and Rivas 1998, p. 97). The leader is, after all, a member of the group. Forsyth (1999, p. 344) describes this well, highlighting those elements of reciprocity, transaction, social exchange and co-operation which characterise the group's interactive process. In some groups, the leader may disclose information or stories which can strengthen the mutuality of members and the leader in ways which help to promote mutual learning (Butler and Wintram 1995, p. 83; Dean 1998, p. 34). Heather comments:

Sometimes we disclose things if we think it's relevant—we don't hold back . . . we do it in a sense of the information we're asking them to disclose, that's the same expectation we have of ourselves . . . self-disclosure is also [a strategy] to contain [the group]—to set the exposure level.

As Benjamin et al. (1997, p. 127) point out: 'facilitation is based on a capacity to manage social relationships. Like any relationship, it cannot work well unless there is reciprocity . . .' Leadership, then, is essentially a shared function which does not belong solely with the designated leader. 'Leadership strategies are comparable to a bag of tools: some are more applicable to certain situations than others . . . such strategies can come . . . just as effectively from those who are designated "members" as from those designated "leaders"' (Douglas 2000, p. 49). For example, in many groups an 'internal leader' emerges, deriving his/her authority both from the reciprocal processes in the group and from those valued abilities and skills that other participants consider him/her to exemplify (Shulman 1999, p. 505). Robyn comments:

People come to the group to learn something from an expert—they look to you (the leader) as the expert—but as the group evolves and they start to get used to the group environment . . . they do find that they do learn from each other in different ways . . . I don't think they come expecting that to happen . . .

Thus leadership is not a static or unchanging phenomenon. Rather, it is a resource available to all members to draw upon and use in order to meet both individual and collective needs. These needs change over the life of the group. As Helen says:

> Leadership is not just a person . . . it isn't encapsulated in an individual but is a series of tasks that anyone can do . . . and then the group has a lot more knowledge and experience available to it . . .

Leadership change

Very importantly, leaders—whether designated or emerging from the membership—need to be able to recognise that at different moments their leadership role may need to be relinquished in order for the group to change and develop. In a critique of an episode of group work, Sullivan (1995, p. 29) notes that a failure by the worker to relinquish control in effect limited the development of the group towards participant autonomy. Such a failure, Sullivan also contends, provides an example of the worker's inability to 'think group' (see Chapter 5). As Butler and Wintram (1995, p. 79) propose: 'Our aim should be to make ourselves (the group leaders) redundant.'

While we will discuss in detail the phases, stages and cycles that characterise groups over time (Chapter 7), it is relevant to note here that leadership acts will differ at different times in the group's life (see, for example, Burkhardt 1982; Sullivan 1995; Nosko and Wallace 1997; McCallum 1997). For example, in the initial stage the leader may need to be more active in structuring the group by promoting the development of particular responses amongst members. Emphasising confidentiality and working to ensure that members bond with each other can be a first step towards developing group cohesion. A group which is cohesive, where members trust each other, is more likely to achieve its purposes without being derailed by frequent absenteeism, silence, antagonism, and so on. Once group members have begun to trust each other, the work of the group can take place. At this point the leader may actively support the emergence of other internal leaders within the group to ensure that the direction pursued is in accord with collective needs. As the group moves towards termination, the leader may take a more assertive role in preparing members for eventual separation and working to ensure that the gains made are able to be sustained. Robyn sums up this changing process well: 'The bonding of the group helps leadership evolve within the group—they feel they've got skills and a knowledge base (by the end of the program) that can equip them.'

Leaderless groups

Some groups are established from the outset to be 'leaderless'—that is, to function without a designated leader. Self-help and advocacy groups are sometimes designed in this way. However, being without a designated leader does not mean that internal leaders will not emerge—indeed, the group is planned so this will occur. Power in such groups belongs with those who, at different times, have more influence over what happens in the group than do others. For example, Bob's group, Men Against Sexual Assault, arose out of and works to exemplify a pro-feminist theoretical stance—that is, a perspective which explains dominant masculinity in structural and cultural terms (see Pease and Camilleri 2001, p. 7). Roles, including that of the leader, are rotated and the group structures itself as a collective rather than a hierarchical entity. Discussions in the group are not led by anyone in particular, but those who are more knowledgable about a particular issue or who have read more widely on the topic are recognised in the group as 'intellectual leaders'. The tasks of leadership—convening meetings, circulating materials and so on—are distributed amongst members and there is active encouragement from members towards newer or less experienced participants taking on leadership tasks.

Where does power come from?

One way to approach the question of where power comes from in the group is to ask what participants bring to the group.

In identifying the various elements that members bring to the group, we will focus discussion on the designated leader or facilitator of the group—usually the person who originates it. However, as has been argued above, all participants will bring aspects of these contributions at different times in the group's life. It is important to appreciate that all participants have contributions to make to the leadership of the group and the direction the group takes as it evolves. Individuals' leadership attributes may be incipent rther than evident at first. Nevertheless, part of the designated leader's role is to nurture and develop these leadership capacities in all participants.

The leader's contribution

The group leader brings a range of resources and qualities to the group. Some of these can be identified as follows:.

Ideas, purposes, theories, visions

- an initial idea for the establishment of a group;
- a purpose which a group is considered to be the best modality to pursue;
- a theoretical or meta-theoretical perspective;
- a vision of what a group can be and can become—what it can achieve;
- an orientation towards the social world in which is embedded values and beliefs about the nature of social reality;
- the anticipation that potential group members will become engaged both with him/her, the other group members and the proposed group purpose.

Structural position

- he/she brings him/herself to the group as a member of society, occupying a particular structural position by virtue of his/her gender, education, economic status, class, ethnicity, ability, sexual orientation;
- resources of authority or position in the auspicing organisation, time, information, knowledge, energy.

Personal dimensions

- personal characteristics such as humour, seriousness, emotional well-being, idiosyncracies;
- a particular style of leading;
- a desire to be a part of something with others, which may also benefit him/herself.

Capabilities

- skills and knowledge which might achieve the group's purpose;
- the capacity to 'think group'.

All of these elements (and perhaps others in addition) in combination, when put to the task of influencing others to bring about change, account for the power which is considered synonymous with group leadership. It is useful to explore them further.

Ideas, purposes, theories and visions

Leadership begins with the idea of establishing a group. Usually the person who originates the idea goes on to set up, and frequently to take a key role in, the group's development. Thus, when one begins to think of establishing a group, one already has in mind a purpose which can best be achieved by a group. In starting out to recruit or invite potential participants to join this group, the originator usually meets on a one-to-one basis with those individuals who could be interested. By doing this, the originator has already taken a leadership role, or may be perceived as having done so by the potential participants. So, well before the first meeting of the group, the leader has identified him/herself as such, either directly or indirectly.

While this process is probably common to the beginning of most groups, the way in which leadership is conceptualised and practised may be very different. As we have discussed in Chapter 2, the specification of purpose refers explicitly to the way in which an issue is problematised, which in turn gives us insight into the theoretical perspective embedded in the type of group formed and the processes likely to characterise it.

Theoretical contributions

In the previous chapter, we reviewed prevailing theories drawn upon for group work from five different vantage points:

- the group as a power base;
- the group as a system;
- the group as container of individuals;
- the group as container of properties;
- the group as a site for meaning construction.

From these, we can logically adduce the kind of leadership, or the different kinds of things which leaders working from these different vantage points might be expected to do. Of course, as groups are established with different theoretical and meta-theoretical bases, there will be differences in the aspects of the group which the leader chooses to focus upon.

- Where the group is conceptualised as a power base, the leader's role is likely to be that of working to develop the potential of members to empower themselves and weld the group into a collectivity which can achieve its change purposes both personally and structurally.

- Where the group is conceptualised as a system, the leader's role is likely to be that of 'system manager', mediating between individuals and the group and other external systems to establish a helping system to benefit all.
- Where the group is conceptualised as comprising individuals, the leader is likely to focus his/her attention on how individuals work together in the group to achieve the individual aims and needs of members collectively, facilitating interpersonal interaction and offering interpretations and information to assist understanding.
- Where the group is conceptualised as a container of properties, the leader's role may be to focus principally on prevailing patterns—of communication, cohesion, culture, development—in order to maximise their effectiveness and minimise their negative impact for the achievement of the collective group purpose.
- Where the group is conceptualised as a site for meaning construction, the leader's role may be to be a participant–observer and facilitator of the group's processes, enabling the sharing and interpretation of stories and narratives.

These different ways in which the leader's role is a function of the purpose and theoretical perspective adopted tell us something of the vision the group leader may hold for the group—for example, that the group will become a site of solidarity and resistance, that it will work in harmony, that individuals will achieve their personal goals, that the group will grow and develop, that it will be a place for the sharing and understanding of subjectivity and identity.

As well as theoretical knowledge, group leaders derive knowledge from a range of sources, including education, training, supervision and wide reading. However one source of particular value for knowing about leading a group is experience—especially that derived from being a participant in a group.

You learn all the time really . . . (Heather)

For years I've lived and worked in groups of men . . . lots of things I've learned there translate into stuff here . . . (Chris)

Helen, who is a member and leader of a social action group, comments:

Unless people have had the experience, it's like talking to people about riding a bicycle . . . you [need to] get yourself into a group . . .

Structural positioning

The leader's power may be 'actual power' and derive from the leader's professional status, education, organisational position and experience. For example, organisational position usually gives the designated leader access to the various tangible resources useful in running a group, such as having suitable accommodation, child care, transport, the availability of time, materials such as photocopying facilities, paper, and so on. All of these are often essential prerequisites for establishing and sustaining a group. In addition, the legitimacy within the agency to establish a group and receive the cooperation necessary from colleagues to do so, for example, by making referrals or tolerating an influx of people, can be crucial to the group's survival.

However, of perhaps even greater significance is the power that is derived from social structures of gender, class and ethnicity. As groups are located within particular social, historical and cultural contexts, they reflect the political and social structures of those contexts. Class, ethnic and gender divisions are the basis for economic and social domination. The person who takes on the leadership role in a group embodies those same structural elements. Without acknowledgment of this and a critical analysis of its impact, a leader may fall into the 'false equality' trap (Butler and Wintram 1995, p. 74) and minimise differences between themselves and participants. A lack of awareness of the structural determinants of power seriously compromises the capacity of the group to function in ways which benefit rather than damage participants. Women in groups, for example, may be very differently positioned in structural terms in relation to their experience of oppression and their possession of knowledge and skills. Their identity as women does not preclude considerable differences in class, race, culture and economics. As Butler and Wintram (1995, p. 75) point out in relation to feminist group work: 'Sisterhood does not mean obscuring the fact that women have different and unequal material circumstances, and acquire knowledge and skills through a range of routes.'

Contributions from feminist theorising and group practice have focused primarily on the importance of women working collectively to achieve personal and social change (Weeks 1994). To this end, feminist writers have offered reconceptualistions of the idea of leadership, recognising that the gender of the leader is highly significant (Rosenberg 1996). Indeed, some feminist writers have argued persuasively that women's groups should be led by women in order to maximise women's sense of safety (especially if they have been victims of violence or sexual abuse), and to assist them to validate their own experience and their own capacity to find answers to their problems. Where groups for women are led by men, it is likely that the group itself will come to replicate the structural inequalities permeating the wider society. (For a fuller discussion of these issues and group work with women experiencing domestic violence, see Rawlings and Carter 1977; Reed and Garvin 1983; Weeks 1988; Brown and Dickey 1992; Schoenholtz-Reed 1996; Shaw et al. 1999; Paroissien and Stewart 2000; Parsons 2001.) The women in the Breast Cancer Therapy Group comment tellingly: 'I think we'd also agree that there's a few things we don't say because he's a male . . . some of the things we say later over coffee . . .'

Men's groups led by men have received relatively little attention. Early work such as Tiger's (1969) took a social Darwinian approach to men's groups, while Hornacek (1977; see also Stein 1983) and others began to rethink men's groups from a pro-feminist perspective. Pease (1988) provides an interesting account of his own journey as a founder and participant in developing theorising and practice of pro-feminist men's groups. The leader of a pro-feminist men's group requires an awareness of the 'pull' towards collusion against women that can be the legacy of men's structural domination. While the assertive pro-feminist agenda may heighten participants' sensitivity to collusion, 'the downside of it is that we struggle to find ways of connecting with each other as men that are not at the expense of women . . .' (Bob)

Co-leading

Co-leadership is frequently the preferred practice adopted by group workers (see Kahn 1996). The choice to work in this way is predicated on the establishment of an effective partnership which may model for group participants the process of 'visible differences working in harmony' (Douglas 2000, p. 58). Co-leaders offer the group different frames of reference and ways of working. The opportunity is available for members to receive input, support and challenge from two different but compatible workers. Here the workers can model the sharing and negotiating of power towards achieving mutually agreed outcomes (see Kahn 1996, p. 443). Chris comments:

> Co-leadership is absolutely essential. You can play tag, or rest in the back pocket and reflect on the process . . . co-leaders model interaction. We challenge each other, joke, we don't necessarily agree—but it takes time to work out how to work together.

And Heather says:

> There's just too much work in a group to do it on your own . . . we dove-tail in quite nicely together.

However, male and female co-leadership can similarly reflect structural gender inequalities which may become apparent in a tendency within the group to devalue or deny the woman co-leader's competence. Further, there may be expectations that the female leader will exemplify caring and emotionally nurturing attributes while the male leader will be expected to exemplify rationality and problem-solving attributes (Schoenholtz-Reed 1996; Nosko and Wallace 1997). Nevertheless, as Rosenberg (1996, p. 438) argues, a male and female co-leader team 'can present the most effective gender role modelling of all'. In goups for men who are violent or sexual abusers, male and female co-leadership has been seen as providing opportunities for the leaders to model non-stereotypic gender relationships. By adopting a shared leadership role, they may both make use of confrontative and supportive interventions. In these kinds of groups, male participants may have the opportunity to explore the point-of-view of women with regard to the impact of their behaviour, as well as having opportunities to develop their capacities to understand and relate to women in less aggressive and oppressive ways (Nosko and Wallace 1997; McCallum 1997; Hall 2001). Co-leadership requires that the leaders work together to establish an effective partnership based on a recognition of the structural features relating to gender and power which impact so significantly on group processes.

Clearly, in all groups, the leader's role must be the object of critical analysis in order to expose differences in terms of power and influence which lie in structural inequalities. As Sachs (1991, p. 189) emphasises, one of the structures which may most need transforming in the group is 'the mind and thinking of the leaders themselves' to enable them to recognise differences in values and beliefs between leaders and participants. He comments (1991, p. 194) that 'all people have power, and through the dialogical process begin to emphasise the freedom to use that power towards ending their own oppression and the oppression of others. Through this process both leaders and people become cooperating subjects in the historical process.'

The group can become the setting for reflection and action on the position of leaders and members. Indeed, it must do so if it is to maximise the potential of all participants, including the leader, to create a site for collective thinking and action. Group leaders require a theoretical and value base which provides them with understanding of the relationship between power and oppression and how these might 'play out' within the group. The ways in which different forms of oppression (class, gender, racial, cultural) interact is complex and the subject of debate. Within the group, this may mean that the leader focuses on ways of assisting group members to explore and analyse power differences, and to ensure that all members take part in decision-making within the group. McLachlan and Reid (1994, p. 59) comment:

> there are always limits on who can say what, under what circumstances, and to whom. Asymmetries in the power relations between people, certain institutional settings, the gender, age, education or ethnicity of the participants in an exchange . . . these are all factors of which we may be only partially aware, but which nevertheless affect not only how we interpret experience but also how, when or even whether we can give expression to our interpretations.

Personal dimensions of leadership

The leader's power to influence may be attributed to him/her by participants—that is, it may come from the members' perception of the leader's ability to lead. Bernard, a group participant, commented:

> He . . . is pretty powerful . . . he's in a powerful position . . . he has to be fairly powerful . . .

And Maria, from a self-help/advocacy group, pointed out:

... a leader must be patient, caring, telling people how well they're doing, drawing people in and keeping them there . . .

The leader as a 'central person', in Douglas's perspective (2000, p. 55) is the one member of the group with whom, in all likelihood, all members have had an initial relationship at the time they considered entry into the group. To this, members may not only attribute power but may also have the expectation that the leader will protect them within the group and be the person to whom they can turn for support. Benjamin et al. (1997, p. 120; see also Corey 2000, pp. 28–32) highlight personal qualities of the facilitator which they suggest are important to bring to the leadership task: self-assurance, an interest in others, a willingness to learn from others, generosity and a healthy self-esteem. Lou comments: 'To be a group leader you have to be fully centred . . . and to a degree resilient . . . there's something potentially very overwhelming in the large group . . .'

Styles of leadership

How the leader influences the processes and directions the group takes is implicit in the style of leadership he/she adopts. The style of leading can also be thought of as a strategy which a leader can shape in ways useful for meeting the group's needs and achieving its purposes. Leadership style is embedded in the leader's theoretical and value base, his/her beliefs about how collective action can be effective in achieving the group's goals and, about how individuals achieve change in their lives, and the belief one has in the group's purpose being to help members achieve change (Toseland and Rivas 1998, p. 121). It will also relate closely with the leader's personal attributes and characteristics.

Leadership styles reflect the leader's conceptualisation of power and his/her beliefs about where power in the group should be located. Thus leadership style will refer to the leader's theoretical orientation and its perceived complimentarity with the participants' needs.

A number of leadership styles have been identified (Byrt 1978; Benjamin et al. 1997).

- An *authoritarian* style locates power in the leaders or facilitators who know what is best for the group. They will direct it, allocating tasks and roles in order to achieve this. In some circumstances—such as a crisis—this may be an appropriate type of leadership.

- A *manipulative* style is adopted by a leader who wishes to dominate the situation but also to take account of the views of others. In the process, he/she tries to sell or structure the situation so that others act as he/she wishes by, for example, filtering or interpreting information. An example of this might be a meeting of a political party. Power is located in the leader and access to it by others may be illusory.

- A *democratic* style of leadership or facilitation will seek participation and collaboration in decision-making and attempt to negotiate and share responsibility across the group. This might occur, for example, in a staff group or a multidisciplinary team of health professionals. This leadership style is characterised by a belief that power will be located in the relationships within the group.

- In *laissez-faire* or *permissive* leadership or facilitation styles, group members are left alone to do as they please. No one is expected to take responsibility for the group; everything depends on the exchange system within the group. An example of this kind of 'free market' group might be a study group. Here power is seen as diffused, with each participant able to exert equal influence on others and on the group as a whole.

Alongside notions of leadership style is the consideration that how the leader is perceived by participants (and by him/herself) may relate closely to gender-based social role stereotyping. This refers to the expectation that males and females will lead groups differently but in ways which conform to sex-role stereotyping. Rosenberg (1996, p. 428), reporting work done at the Tavistock Group Relations Conference, argues that male leaders are associated with an 'agentic' role, characterised by assertiveness, controlling tendencies, independence and personal efficiency. Female leaders are associated with a 'communal' role which is characterised by concern for others, caring, nurturing, interpersonal sensitivity and emotional expressiveness. Because 'communal' characteristics are more often associated with traditional expectations about how women should behave, they are less valued than 'agentic' roles. However, as we saw in our earlier discussion of co-leadership— especially with relation to work with men who are violent—should group leaders subvert this stereotyping by, for example, women leaders taking on more assertive behaviours, the group members' anxiety and anger may be aroused. According to Wright and Gould (1996, p. 338), research indicates that female leaders will evoke even more powerfully negative reactions than male leaders should they be perceived to have adopted a non sex-role stereotypic leadership style.

Capability

It is understandable that beginning group leaders often approach group work with considerable anxiety. As Lou notes, 'it takes a fair amount of robustness to get up and feel that you can facilitate'. This anxiety is in part due to their recognition that they are likely to be seriously outnumbered. This can be a threatening realisation. It is worth remembering that many group members may feel the same, especially on joining a group. Other sources of anxiety emphasised by beginning group leaders—and not restricted to them—refer to how the leader works with participants who may be perceived as difficult or disruptive—perhaps those who are silent or those who dominate— and the emergence of conflict and disagreement in the group. A leader may react by exerting strict control over the group, thereby inhibiting rather than working with the group (Sullivan 1995; see also Mondros and Berman-Rossi 1991 in relation to community development groups). However, knowing how to deal with the unexpected (and the expected) is a powerful contribution made (initially at least), by the group leader. It comes from the leader's ongoing experience, grounded in theoretical knowledge, an understanding of individuals' particular circumstances and an awareness of the power of the group itself.

Clearly, to lead a group requires a particular kind of capability. In my conversations with leaders and participants, some of the following reflections on what is needed to lead a group well were identified. They also demonstrate the connection between the group's theoretical base and the kind of leading that goes with it:

> You need skills to balance the content and the process. For me it's a constant challenge to filter out what's the most valuable information and how I can present it in a way that gets the most impact in the short time I have . . . (Robyn, psychoeducational group)

> I think [the leader] has a pretty good knowledge of each member of the group and what their situation is, and I think he's acting strategically in relation to each of them . . . I'm sure he has each particular person's position in mind, where they're coming from . . . (Bernard, psychotherapy group)

> [The leader needs to] actually show them how they can respond differently and how they can help each other by supporting that change . . . (Chris, behaviour change group for men who are violent)

> You need the leader/facilitator/therapist who's going to hold it all together and allow all that [emotion] to sit safely . . . (Lou, large psychotherapy/psychoeducational group)

> We try [to] externalise all those issues people experience and talk about strategies about how to deal with them . . . (Heather, support and psychoeducational group)

I need a bit of an intimate idea of the strengths and weaknesses of each member so I can really get maximum consciousness out of the group . . . (Cynthia, support and therapy group for mothers with terminal illness, and their children)

You've got to be really clear what you're trying to achieve when you set up and then be prepared to modify it . . . (Helen, social action group)

Many of those writing on the topic of leadership in groups specify or list the range of skills required. Douglas (2000, p. 48), for example, identifies the skills leaders contribute as 'guidance, enabling and direction' and terms them 'leadership acts'. He comments further (2000, p. 57) that:

a process of guiding, of encouraging, of sharing the consequences of behaviour patterns and of asking whether this is what was intended; of making visible behaviour which is beginning to show understanding of what is required and of deflecting the effects of bad behaviour to protect those liable to be hurt, but always making specifically clear what is going on.

Very similar leadership skills are identified by Butler and Wintram (1995, p. 84) in their discussion of feminist group work.

Toseland and Rivas (1998, p. 104) also identify three groups of skills the leader brings to the task:

• facilitating group processes by such actions as involving members, focusing the group's communication and clarifying the content which is emerging;
• data gathering and assessment—this requires the leader to ensure that members' thoughts and feelings are understood by requesting information or asking questions;
• action—at times the group leader may provide support or

challenge and confront members to assist them in moving forward in tackling and resolving the difficulties they encounter.

To these we might add the leader's conceptual and organisational skills, which are evident in the clarity with which the group's purpose is articulated and the process through which the group plans to achieve it.

Many other writers on the topic of group leadership offer somewhat prescriptive accounts of the skills needed to lead a group. Generally, these are divided into task and process (or group maintenance) skills (Benson 1987; Spence and Goldstein 1995; Forsyth 1999, Ch. 12; Shulman 1999, Chs 2 and 13). Task skills refer to what the leader does in order to 'get things done'—for example, assist members to make decisions, set time frames and boundaries around the group, enforce guidelines for acceptable behaviour, and so on. Maintenance, or process, skills refer to those which are directed towards building and strengthening the interpersonal layer of group life so that the group's tasks can be done and the purposes achieved. Maintenance skills would include such things as offering support and encouragement, helping participants talk to one another, managing conflict constructively, focusing on ensuring that participants feel safe and are beginning to develop cohesive relationships in order to experience a sense of solidarity, and offering interpretations about what things mean. Clearly, a combination of both task and maintenance skills is important for group leaders and participants to develop.

For the most part, however, leadership skills have been studied in the abstract because, as many writers argue, they are of general relevance for work with all groups (see Benson 1987; Douglas 2000; Ivey et al. 2001). This is both an advantage and a limitation. It is quite possible to describe and list a range of ways of 'doing' group work, albeit with examples demonstrating the particular skills in action. However, the limitation of this is that knowledge about how to acquire and use these particular skills remains abstracted from practice. Anyone who has been in a group will tell of the considerable fluidity, dynamism, confusion and complexity of that experience—not to mention the emotional and intellectual shifts and turbulence that come with it. Knowing what to do means knowing how to act and how to 'go on' in a situation that is pressurised and demanding. In such circumstances particular skills are certainly required but cannot always be planned for. Rather, most group workers are well able to describe in retrospect what they did or said and why, and sometimes it is the unexpected nature of what they did or said and why it *worked* that they seek to understand.

Although knowing what skills are required is useful, learning about how to lead groups comes most meaningfully from experience and reflection on experience (see Berger 1996; Zastrow 2001). However, in order to learn from and use our experience of being in a group, group workers need to acquire a conceptual frame or cognitive schema to take with them into the group. It is a first priority for a group worker to develop the capacity to always maintain a stance towards the group-as-a-whole, informed by an orientation to discovering what is happening in the group and how it can be understood and shaped towards fulfilling the group's espoused or emerging purpose. This is what is meant by 'thinking group', and it will be the subject of the next chapter.

Summary

In this chapter we have discussed group leadership in relation to issues of power, reciprocity and resources. It was argued that leadership is best understood as inhering in the relationships amongst all group participants, including the designated leader. The various sources that leaders can draw on to establish and maintain their power were described, as were issues of leadership type and style. The chapter ended with a discussion of the kinds of elements that go into making a capable leader—a topic to be developed further in the next two chapters.

5

'THINKING GROUP':
'It's got a life of its own'

In the previous chapter we focused on the contributions which designated leaders and group participants bring to the group. While leading undoubtedly calls on a range of skills, we concluded by arguing that, while the kinds of skills can be listed and described, knowing how to 'do' group work comes from a process of experience and reflection, informed by theoretical and practical knowledge. The point being made in this chapter is that, in order for a group worker to work well, he/she needs to approach their practice—and the group—with a cognitive and emotional frame encompassing the group-as-a-whole. This is what is meant by 'thinking group'.

In order to understand this concept, let us consider the cognitive and emotional transformation that would occur in the following scenario:

> You enter a lift to go from the ground to the fifth floor where your office is located. There are (you haven't counted them) several others in the lift. The door closes and the lift moves off. Then it stops between floors. All at once you are not in a lift conveying you

anywhere: you are in a cramped space which you need to escape from! The individuals sharing the space begin to reveal who they are—men, women, frightened, humorous, English-speakers, students, visitors to the building. Suddenly, rather than anonymous 'others', they start to become allies—you have just formed a group which has a task . . .

In this example, a shared, rather anxiety-provoking external event has transformed your mental frame: you now see a collection of individuals as a group to which you belong, which shares a common predicament and calls for collective action. Of course, the circumstances surrounding the formation of a social group with a purpose which you have originated or joined is somewhat different. Nevertheless, you do have a particular group-based cognitive schema already in place, though it is often not articulated. In Chapter 3, we discussed the various ways groups have been theorised. These theoretical formulations were predicated on a particular way of seeing what a group is and what it can become: a power base, a system, an entity comprising individuals, an entity containing properties, a site of meaning construction. Each of these ways of defining what a group is brings with it a set of possible structures and imperatives for how one works collectively.

Thus, when a group worker works, it is from this basis of an orientation towards, or a mental map of, the group-as-a-whole. So, rather than specifying particular skills and tools for working, it may be more useful to talk about how one develops or constructs such an orientation towards the group-as-a-whole. This is summed up in the invocation to 'think group!'

Thinking group

'Thinking group' means focusing on the group as a whole—considering everything that happens in terms of the group context (also the wider context in which it is embedded—social, economic, political, organisational) because this is where meaning is manifest. This exhortation to 'think group' (attributed to Middleman in Papell 1997; see also Sullivan 1995, p. 28) provides a central orientation point for a group leader. Indeed, it underscores a worker's decision to set up a group with a purpose in mind that is best achieved by the combined forces of a number of individuals. It also emphasises the difference between practice with groups and practice with individuals. Practice with groups is *not* the same as working with several individuals in a group. Rather, group work is, by definition, working with a group.

This distinction is an essential one: when a number of people come together to work on something—increasing their self-esteem, undertaking a task, learning something, changing something—what develops may be characterised as being beyond what occurs when individuals separately try to achieve the same outcome. This is, of course, precisely why a group forms, or was formed, in the first place. In advocating for the group worker to 'think group' we are referring to the necessity for the group worker to keep in mind that, while groups are comprised of individuals, at the same time their coming together may enable the expression of powerful forces reinforcing a sense of commonality and solidarity. These are the building blocks for the development of trust. Trust, and its counterpart—reciprocity amongst members, may establish the bonds which serve to enable members to achieve their individual and common goals. The task of the group worker is to nurture such developments. By 'thinking group' rather then 'thinking individuals', the group worker positions him/herself to see and enhance these elements for the well-being of the whole. This capacity to 'think group' is of central importance across the range of different kinds of groups—psychotherapy, psychoeducational, mutual aid, social action. Mondros and Berman-Rossi's (1991, p. 204) comment in regard to community development groups could apply equally to all groups: 'organisers invite trouble for themselves if they don't attend to . . . the meaning of *group* experience for individuals and matters of group process [emphasis added]'.

To illustrate: an individual's decision to participate in a group is usually accompanied by some ambivalent feelings. Most of us know from our everyday life experiences that groups can be difficult and conflict-ridden enterprises. So a decision to enter one may bring with it a degree of fear and trepidation. Sometimes this ambivalence emerges in silent, angry or withdrawn behaviours. In 'thinking group', the group worker will be attuned to the emergence (often simultaneously) of warm, friendly, open, mistrustful and aggressive behaviours amongst participants. It is his/her task to recognise and understand this ambivalence and, by making it apparent to group participants through comment and interpretation, allowing it to be discussed and worked with. In 'thinking group', the group worker sees everything that happens within and between group participants as 'grist to the mill', part and parcel of the work of the group. Thus the experience of ambivalence itself can be recognised as one of the group's 'raw materials' which needs to be turned into a resource that the group, individually and collectively, can draw upon and build up.

As another example, we might note that it is not uncommon for a particular individual in a group to be scapegoated—that is, to be seen as the source of problems and difficulties. In 'thinking group', the group worker might understand this as a phenomenon characteristic of the group—the desire to remove the bad from individuals by dumping it on one person who then exits (literally or figuratively), taking the bad with him/her. By drawing this dynamic to the attention of the group-as-a-whole, individuals have the opportunity to recognise what is happening, to see the ways in which individuals in the group may want to distance themselves from acknowledging their own flaws, and thus develop a more realistic and tolerant attitude, not only to the 'scapegoat' but also to themselves.

The capacity to 'think group' is the single most important contribution group workers bring to their practice. Group workers are not there to work with individuals *except* through the medium of the group. The group worker's primary goal is to evoke, nurture and harness the collective strengths of group members so they may become a resource to themselves and to one another. The capacity to 'think group' is one way of grasping the meaning of the group experience for all participants, including the group leader. It is also fundamentally involved in the process of interpreting, or making sense of this meaning (both conscious and unconscious), so that it can serve to aid the participants' understanding of themselves, of themselves in relation to others, and in relation to the purpose which underlies the group's existence.

The practice of 'thinking group'

How does the group worker 'think group'? The answer to this question is that they can't avoid doing so. The group worker sets out with the decision to establish a group—presumably because a group was considered the best way of achieving the purpose they had in mind. Again, in these recent conversations I had with group leaders and participants, some of the following comments were made about the decision as to why a group was the best way to achieve the desired purpose:

> Relational identity: rather than constructing a sense of self around separation, you construct a sense of self in relation to others. Hence dialogue is a key issue—dialogues across difference . . . you open up issues with [others] . . . (Bob)

> The group offers a whole different sounding board for the experience or the issue. (Lou)

> Why would you do it on your own? (Helen)

> I was looking down the barrel—I thought I'd be dead by next Christmas, so to hear people who'd lived for three or four years by then seemed to me like a miracle—so I found that part of the group very encouraging. (Breast Cancer Therapy Group)

It empowers people to know that somebody else—[other] people—want to be normal. It's good to find out that those negative feelings you had, [that] everyone's having them, because then they don't become those monsters you have to keep secret . . . you've got another avenue to express [them] and to learn how to deal with it. (Maria)

You really do feel for the other people in the group, even though they're complete strangers to you and you don't socialise with them outside . . . you nevertheless develop this bond and when somebody seems to be handling things better or they have a success or they describe how they've got a job when they've been struggling or something—there's a dynamic there that's difficult to put into words. There's something there—that's what the power of it is. (Bernard)

These quotations demonstrate that the decision to set up or to participate in a group presupposes a concept of the group as-a-whole—an entity, a phenomenon, an experience, a 'thing in itself'. To keep this concept constantly in mind is what is meant by 'thinking group'.

Other 'evidence' for the group worker starting out from a 'thinking group' frame is found in the physical arrangements most often provided for the group meetings. Groups are usually formed in a circle with people facing each other, and in so doing, marking the boundaries. The group circle is like a frame: people look inwards and in relation to others. The circle provides a reflective intersubjective space between people. It seems reasonable to propose that this kind of physical use of space suggests a pre-existing conceptualisation of the group-as-a-whole.

We can also learn more and 'think group' better if we look at the works of others in different domains who are 'thinking group'. Artists who depict groups, for example, use the composition of a group as a means of conveying beliefs, ideas and emotions that have universal resonance. Many of us are familiar with the work of painters such as Botticelli, with his numerous religious and mythological paintings, or Breughel (see front cover illustration) with his scenes of peasants and village life. William Carlos Williams took several of Breughel's paintings as his source of inspiration in creating poems, capturing in words the essence of these painted groups—the emotion, the colour, movement and vitality expressed in people's collective work and celebration (Williams 1976, pp. 211–18).

Painters (and here too poets) use the group as a way of constructing and illuminating the meaning of varied yet specific human experiences. There is, of course, an important difference from social or therapeutic groups and groups depicted in paintings. With our groups, the group worker and the participants create meaning through their co-construction of the group while the artist constructs the group in order to create a meaning which is already in their mind or emerges as they paint or write. As group workers, we create and co-construct meaning from the group in its entirety. The meaning is already contained within the group, or will emerge over time, and our task is to grasp it. In so doing, we are practitioner–theorists, working at the synthesis of theory and practice.

But what is shared in common between group workers and those who paint or poeticise groups is the notion of there being something created which emerges from the poetic, the felt and the imaginary. And, in order to 'think group', the group worker needs to recognise and explore these poetic and imaginary domains. Middleman and Goldberg (1985, p. 5) provide an example: 'What if the worker imagined the group to be actors on a stage? Attention would be attuned to such things as who is upstaging whom, who is out of character, what is the play for the day, who are the main characters, and who are the extras.'

I commented in Chapter 3 that, as group workers, we are often very preoccupied with theoretical constructs for understanding our observations and experience. With this comes a tendency to oppose these theoretical and scientific understandings with 'lived experience'—the poetic, the felt and the imaginary. This is a false dichotomy: in the social sciences where group work belongs, our theories inevitably spring from metaphors. In fact, all theories in the human sciences refer to, derive from or can be traced back to a particular metaphor, or series of metaphors, about the nature of social reality. So, when we come to understanding in this 'poetic' way, when we try to grasp the meaning of the group as a whole as an entity, the way we do it best is via metaphor. Metaphor is central to theory. Burke (quoted in Sapir and Croker 1977, p. 35; see also Adams 1997; Polombo 1996) comments: 'Every perspective requires a metaphor, implicit or explicit, for its organizational base.' Ross (1993, p. 152), notes: 'Metaphor is not merely a linguistic mode of expression; rather, it is one of the chief cognitive structures by which we are able to have coherent, ordered experiences that we can reason about and make sense of.' Metaphor, then, is central to the capacity to construct meaning—a very important capacity of the group worker. And the construction of meaning is what theory development and use is all about. So, when we 'think group', we are simultaneously 'thinking metaphor'.

What is Metaphor?

Gregory Bateson, in conversation with Fritjof Capra (1988, p. 77), comments: 'Metaphor is right at the bottom of being alive.' Roland Barthes (1989, p. 278) argues that metaphor sustains any discourse which asks: 'What is it? What does it mean?'

Metaphors are paradoxical: they enhance our understanding and experience of one kind of thing in terms of another. For example, as those I spoke to said: 'the group is an organism . . . the group is like another family'. Indeed, the group can be all sorts of things to participants at the same time: a gathering of friends, a source of feedback, a tutorial (see Sunderland 1997/98, p. 132). Metaphors assert that something abstract is something concrete and in this way obliquely establish or construct the meaning inherent in the situation. Another way of saying this is that abstract concepts—those building blocks of theory—cannot remain at an abstract level: in practice situations, they need to be rooted in the concrete. Indeed, it is this interplay of these two disparate terms (group—organism; group—another family) which provides us with insight into the meaning or truth value of something (Sapir and Crocker 1997, p. 32; Sunderland 1997/98; Adams 1997). Additionally, as Sunderland (1997/98) points out, when metaphors are revealed they can be used by group workers to change ideas, enabling phenomena to be seen and understood differently. For example:

In a group which normally comprises twelve people including two co-leaders, the chairs are set in a circle. One particular meeting began with only four members arriving on time. These four sat beside the co-leaders, so we were occupying a semi-circle, looking at the empty chairs. One of the co-leaders commented, 'it seems like we are all waiting at the bus stop, waiting for the bus to arrive'. The participants laughed and one of them said she felt more like she was at the theatre, waiting for the curtain to go up. This led to a discussion about waiting on other people as though they were always more important, and that things could not get underway without their presence.

In Chapter 1 we discussed the difficulties of even defining what a group is. At that point I suggested that my preferred definition of a group referred to 'bounded social experience' of some kind. To have used the concept of bounded experience, we have already invoked the metaphor of a boundary—a metaphor which has been prominent in research and theorising in many domains (Petronio et al. 1998): communications theory, family theory, ecological (person—environment) theory, systems theory. This boundary metaphor creates an image of relationships, a sense of being 'within' and 'outside' the boundary, evoking perhaps a sense of the tension that exists between integration and separation, and serving to set the conditions for the development of a group identity.

Thus, by using the metaphor of 'group as bounded social experi-ence', I have already classified groups as being particular kinds of phenomena with particular issues of relevance—for example, the definition of boundaries, the role of boundaries in sustaining or inhibiting interaction, the relationship of the group to the outside world, and so on. Even by naming a collection of individuals as a group we are, in some important sense, naming and identifying this phenomenon and thus prefiguring some kind of response to it. Further, in forming the group into a circle we are working metaphor-ically. On a practical level, the circle enables everyone to see and hear each other, but this can also be achieved by a triangle, parallel lines, a square, an oblong. The circle, however, is metaphorical language for many possible phenomena: for communication, non-hierarchical communication, the enclosure of space, the containment of space, a boundary, people looking inward not outward, and so on.

In previous chapters we have looked at the metaphors other group theorists invoke when they conceptualise the group—a system, a power base, a container, a site for meaning construction. Each of these theories proceeds from a central image and with that comes different kinds of imperatives for understanding and action. For example, the use of consciousness-raising in a social action group may be an impor-tant facet of building a power base (see Butler and Wintram 1995), or the telling of stories may serve to forge and share a sense of one's identity in a therapeutic story-making group (see Gersie 1997).

While this theoretical knowledge underpins the group worker's viewpoint, in 'thinking group' they are also on the alert to identify the images contained in the interactions of group participants. Every group meeting is different and, while this gives group gatherings their dynamism, it also has the potential to overwhelm. Observing from a 'think group' stance allows the group worker to be aware of the dif-ference of each meeting while simultaneously searching to identify the particular image that reveals the central elements of the situation. Middleman and Goldberg (1985, p. 7) comment:

it is the central image, or pattern, that enables the group worker to see the particular group situation as a *kind* of group situation, a special case of a more general type. It is that connection that gives meaning to the particular through isolation and identification of the central image, which produces what we call 'understanding'.

For example, in a group of people who are undergoing treatment for cancer, one member—Max—tells of his radiotherapy, describing it as a visit to the secret offices of MI5. The radiotherapy treatment room is located in the hospital basement, beneath street level. Here staff wear special uniforms, speak a technical language and everything is operated by computers. As Max tells it in the group, others laugh and play with his ideas, elaborating them and celebrating his ingenuity.

In this example, group members refer to their experience in meta-phorical terms. These metaphors bring together ideas that are not literally alike (radiotherapy and MI5). However, when the group worker draws out the meaning that is implied, this may reveal new or different ways of thinking about treatment. So, for example, the awfulness of radiotherapy is being likened to an adventure into the unknown and mysterious territory which is frightening but simultaneously allows the person experiencing it to reframe it in a way which offers the capacity for emotional control in the situation and, with this, the release of creative energies to think and to imagine. Exploring the metaphor and the image 'reveals new possibilities for consideration' (Sunderland 1997/98, p. 132). Max's ideas have become something that all group members can use to help them manage and explore the 'other side' of their situation and share with others who know and understand inti-mately what they are talking about.

Summary

When we 'think group', we are engaging with the 'lived experiences' of leader and participants, with the poetic and the felt. We express our thoughts and ideas by using metaphors. These poetic and imaginative responses are our attempts to construct meaning.

When the group worker is working, he or she may be asking: 'What kind of group is being thought here?' 'What does this group mean?' 'What is happening here?' Asking these questions helps to elicit, on the level of metaphor, the conceptual frameworks we are using. This is one of the ways we as group workers—sometimes consciously and sometimes unconsciously—become theorists in action. We observe, we question and we respond by attempting to understand what may be happening in the group; and we try to account for this by employing working hypotheses and testing them out against our existing experiences as group leaders and/or participants. So, when we 'think group' and try to grasp hold of the metaphors present in the visual and verbal cues coming from the group, we engage our imaginative selves.

When group workers work, they have found a way of integrating their theoretical understanding with the 'lived experience' of facilitating a group. Their capacity to 'think group' has enabled them to make use of the abstract understanding generated through theory in a way which guides and structures their practice. One of the ways the group worker in action weaves between the scientific, the felt and the poetic, the theoretical and the practical is by means of metaphor. Metaphors emerge best when we 'think group'. Very importantly, the act of interpretation and meaning construction places our focus squarely on process: what is happening here and now and what it might mean. To stay with and try to understand the process whereby meaning is being constructed as events unfold is a capacity of central importance to practitioners. In fact, practice cannot be taken as a 'given'; rather, it is a set of developing processes. This means that we are constantly working as theorists. We all know from our practice experience that no static theory is adequate to the task of capturing the fluidity and chameleon-like character of human interaction, always synonymous with change and uncertainty. We need a frame to view it through: this is what is meant by 'thinking group'.

6

'THINKING GROUP' IN ACTION:
'Dealing with the dynamics of a very emotional thing'

'Thinking group' is, in essence, the adoption of a conceptual frame for approaching the practice of group work. However, group workers also need to develop various action strategies and techniques to allow them to put the 'thinking group' frame into practice. In this chapter we will identify and discuss six such action strategies:

- participating and observing;
- listening;
- remembering;
- thinking;
- speaking;
- contextualising—or working with diversity.

Participating and Observing

Critical to the capacity to 'think group' is the group worker's ability to be a competent participant observer. Douglas (2000, p. 48; see also Dean 1998) argues that this is a fundamental skill brought to the group by the leader. Participating and observing mean developing the capacity to observe people in the group and to note what is taking place, to be particularly attuned to the less obvious visual and linguistic cues expressed in metaphor. Leaders, then, are skilled participant–observers. Such a stance might appear contradictory unless we bear in mind that participating and observing occur as if on a continuum. The participant may move from being a 'complete participant'—that is, being absorbed into the group—to a 'complete observer'—that is, almost entirely detached. In practice, however, skilled workers move up and down this continuum, moving in and out of the group as the process unfolds. Such a stance enables them to register their emotional and empathic responses in order to understand and communicate the meaning they interpret to the group.

To be able to participate and observe is very important, both in order to know what is going on in the group and in order to be a witness to what is happening. By witnessing an event, we are giving recognition and ascribing meaning and validation to the importance of what is happening. In Bridget's group, the Women's Circus, the presence of an audience is highly significant. She comments:

If we don't do a performance, which is having an audience, then we would turn more on ourselves and lose energy . . . you have to have a solution if there's an audience—be inventive, think on your feet, be responsible for what you do . . . there's no hiding . . .

While very few of the groups with which human service workers work perform for an outside audience, the significance of speaking or confessing or expressing emotions and feelings in the presence of two or more people is a highly charged event. In fact, it is often the source of considerable fear amongst group participants. Nevertheless, participants frequently report on the catharsis and relief that follow their ability to confide in those around them whose presence as observers and witnesses who are simultaneously participants can generate. Robyn notes:

group members will almost always comment that there's something about the richness they get from being with other people in the same situation—the normalising of their experience as a human experience—that is the most powerful thing . . .

What do we observe?

There is always so much going on in a group that it is important to bear in mind some of the following events or phenomena on which we might focus our observations:

- what we can see: both verbal and non-verbal behaviours—for example, that someone is silent but absorbed in the group conversation; that someone is upset or tearful; that someone has pushed their chair back outside the group circle; that someone decides to leave the room at a particularly tense moment;
- our own physical, emotional or bodily reactions to what is happening—for example, that we are starting to feel annoyed; that we are looking at our watch; that we are thinking about what we will do after the groups ends.

What do we 'do' with our observations?

Our first task is to note what we have observed. We then must try to make some sense of our observations in relation to the group-as-a-whole, and in relation to the group's purpose. We might ask ourselves questions—for example: Why Am I looking at my watch? Am I bored? Anxious? What does this tell me about what might be going on here? For example, might this mean that the group-as-a-whole is bored, or is wanting to avoid some difficult issues that could be emerging?

Listening

The group leader's capacity to listen empathically in a way informed by his/her theoretical knowledge is closely allied to the practice of participant observation and is another component of 'thinking group'. Corradi-Fiumara (1990) argues that most of us know how to speak, but few know how to listen. She refers to listening as 'the other side of language', asserting that the activity of listening provides an opportunity for cooperative creativity. Quoting from Heidegger, she notes (1990, p. 174) that if we succeed in hearing what language really says when people speak, 'then it may happen—provided we proceed carefully—that we get more truly to the matter that is expressed in any talking and asking'. When referring to the leaders in their group, the women in the Breast Cancer Therapy Group noted: 'They have to learn to listen and know when to come in—that's not easy to do . . . it needs lots of compassion.' Helen comments in relation to her social action group:

> You need to be able to listen to what the people in the group are saying . . . you have to listen very carefully not just to what's being said but to what's being meant because somehow people say something and sometimes the words don't carry the meaning . . .

Chris echoes this: 'They [the men in the group] are going to be listened to respectfully, they're going to be listened to and heard . . .' Gersie (1997, p. 204), referring to her work with Therapeutic Storymaking Groups, emphasises the necessity for participants and the leader to pay attention to developing their listening capacities—'listening to one's listening'—in order to enhance communicative clarity and the healing effect that comes with the feeling that 'someone else has understood'.

Listening, then, is central to the group worker's practice but it is a skill which sometimes tends to be taken for granted. We need to ask: how do we know what to listen to, what to listen for and what constitutes 'good' listening? Here are some guidelines:

Listening to

The group worker begins by listening to what is being said, the content or issue being talked about and the language, words or metaphors the speaker chooses in order to express him/herself. The worker might then ask him/herself:

- to whom is the speaker speaking—to a particular individual? To the group-as-a-whole? To no one in particular? To him/herself?
- what does it mean for the group-as-a-whole and this person (the speaker) to be speaking to these listeners at this time? What sense or meaning might I make of this?

With these questions, the worker is trying to listen to and understand both the speaker's communication and elements of the meta-communication (the communication about the communication) that accompany it. The worker listens in this way in order to grasp the meaning being communicated which has resonance both for the person speaking and for the group-as-a-whole. Grasping what is being communicated tells the worker a great deal about what is happening in the group and how well the purposes of the group-as-a-whole are being achieved.

Listening for

The group worker also listens for:

- what is *not* being said, which may indicate that certain issues are being avoided or are not yet ready to be spoken about—perhaps because they are perceived as dangerous or uncomfortable;
- themes which begin to emerge over time as the group returns to what appear to be continuing preoccupations. For example, in a social support group for people with a chronic illness, the themes of food, cooking and eating continually reappeared. In hearing these themes, the worker may want to explore with the group

what they mean and why they have such importance to the group-as-a-whole;

- ways in which the worker's theoretical perspective may enhance the understanding of what is being listened to. For example, a worker with a psychoanalytic frame might listen for or be prompted to hear more clearly, ideas, words or metaphors that suggest concepts of particular significance to 'psychoanalytic ears'. The same ideas, words or metaphors may not be heard quite so clearly by a worker whose focus is on listening for the group participants' readiness to take political action.

What is 'good' listening?

It is difficult to be prescriptive about what constitutes 'good' listening. However, perhaps a useful way of judging the quality of listening is in relation to its effects. Does one's listening, when it is 'translated' into the spoken word (see below), enable the group-as-a-whole to move ahead in achieving its purposes?

'Good' listening requires the worker to frequently remain silent in order to hear what is being said. It is something of a truism to state that we can't talk and listen at the same time with any degree of confidence that we are still able to hear what is going on. Some workers describe their listening to be rather like sitting in a train watching the scenery pass by—that is, they are attending to what is happening (listening) but not jumping too quickly into stating categorically what they have heard. Rather, they remain in the present, monitoring and absorbing the passing scene of words, images and ideas and, bit by bit, increasing their understanding of what they are hearing.

Remembering

To remember what has been happening over time within the group-as-a-whole, as well as for individual participants, is a key component of 'thinking group'. To have the capacity to remember is sometimes taken for granted, but it remains an important strategy in group work for several reasons.

Remembering suggests that the worker is keeping in mind both the group-as-a-whole and the individual participants' various journeys over the life of the group. To actively keep something in mind is to provide a very containing and supportive role in the group. Groups, as we know, can be turbulent, highly charged and sometimes very confusing and overwhelming places, both for the worker and for the participant. In this environment, the act of remembering helps to retain focus and stability. It can be very helpful and affirming for someone's behaviour or contribution to the group to be remembered, and at times recalled. This act may be effective in establishing a sense of identity and substance for both the group-as-a-whole and for individual participants. (There are parallels here, of course, in the ways in which nations celebrate or confirm their collective identities by remembering and recording their histories. Family photograph albums perform the same function.)

How does the group worker remember?

The capacity to remember can be strengthened in various ways. For example, some workers make a deliberate effort to remember the first and the final words that are said at each group meeting. They find that this helps them later recall with ease the bits that came in between. Others write notes immediately after a meeting. To work with a co-leader increases the amount of material that is remembered, provided that time is spent together at the end recalling and recording the meeting (see Chapter 10).

What to remember?

The kinds of elements that might be important to remember include:

• key themes or preoccuations of the meeting;

- any unusual behaviour of participants;
- the apparent impact of any comments the worker(s) made;
- any previously unknown information that emerged;
- anything that was *not* said or did *not* happen that the worker(s) might have expected would be done or said.

Thinking

The concept and the practice of 'thinking group' provide a short-hand expression for finding a cognitive schema and a practice orientation that maximises the group worker's capacity to think in action. Group work practitioners, perhaps even more than one-to-one workers, are faced with the potentially overwhelming complexity which is synonymous with a group. 'Thinking group' is one way of enabling the group worker to manage their own involvement with the group. Some of the complexity encountered in the group arises from the contradictory nature of the group leader's positioning. He or she is required to be both participant and observer, both insider and outsider; the leader's role requires the setting of limits and boundaries at the same time as it requires him/her to encourage experimentation and risk-taking; to create a sense of stability at the same time as the group's purpose is to work towards change. Being able to work in and with contradictions requires the capacity to recognise and cope with complexity. Such a capacity is potentially very powerful, and must be crafted carefully towards the benefit of the group and its participants. Group work is demanding emotionally and physically, and is always unpredictable— 'It challenges your own sense of life, or generosity, or struggle.' (Chris)

A particular challenge which group workers face is that of thinking under pressure. In a group, such pressure might come in the form of competing demands from participants, emotionally charged encounters, confusion, not knowing what is going on—in fact, the very scenario where a clear-thinking approach is likely to be essential! To be able to think means being able to maintain a focus and a connection to

the purpose the group has been set up to meet. We have already discussed in greater detail the exhortation to 'think group!' (see Chapter 5)
and this remains the basic frame from within which the worker acts. It
is not always easy to maintain this frame, but it can become something
like a 'default' position if we find we are beginning to feel overwhelmed.
The questions posed in the previous chapter are relevant here:

• What kind of a group is happening here?
• What does this group mean at this moment?

When we try to answer these questions we think about various
possible explanations for making sense of what we are experiencing
and hearing. These possible explanations are derived from what
we know theoretically and from previous experience. The group
worker's thinking in the group may take the form of play—playing
with possible ideas and images, turning them this way and that until
we find a way of putting things together which provides a coherent
explanation. Having or providing an explanation for something or
some feelings which seem bewildering can be a powerful influence
which can both stabilise and move the group forward towards
meeting its purposes—be they insight or political action or behaviour control.

How does the group worker think in action?

This is a perennial and complex question with which probably all
practitioners grapple; a topic to which writers such as Schon (1983),
Ixer (1999), Taylor and White (2000), and Thompson (2000) have
contributed important insights. While we do not have the scope here
to explore this question in any depth, two points are noteworthy. The
first is the centrality of working from a 'thinking group' frame, as we
have already discussed. The second is that each group worker would
do well to set time aside to explore his/her own preferred or usual way
of working, to ask the following:

- Do I usually act and then think about why I did something?
- Do I usually think first and then take action?
- In which situations do I do either of these in that sequence?

Trying to answer these questions may provide a useful point of departure for considering the efficacy of one's thinking-in-action and the conditions which facilitate or inhibit either thinking or acting.

All group workers benefit from opportunities to debrief and to think critically about their work. Various approaches to supervision and models of critical reflection have arisen from different theoretical and practice perspectives. Theory and practice interweave in complex and not always well-understood ways, but it remains of considerable importance to the development of both that ways are found to integrate them, in order—as Thompson (2000) suggests— to 'get at the knowledge which is in the action'. 'Thinking group' is one such strategy.

Speaking

When the group worker says something in the group, he or she will most likely be making a significant impact, and this should not be under-estimated. Its significance lies in the fact that what is said is the culmination and expression in words of all the previous actions we have been describing—participating and observing, listening, remembering and thinking. The form of words chosen and their purposes are highly strategic—that is, they are (on some level) planned in order to achieve something—a change in thinking or understanding, in emotions or feelings, in behaviour or comprehension, whether focused on an individual participant or the group-as-a-whole.

In essence, whenever the group worker speaks, he or she is offering an interpretation of some kind. The words used are interpretive— that is, they provide a meaning of some kind, about something, for someone. These interpretations may be any or all of the following:

101

- empathic comments aimed at drawing out or exploring feelings and emotions;
- clarifying comments to ensure that what someone has said is what they intended to say;
- engaging comments to invite participants to join in;
- challenging or confronting comments which might highlight contradictions or identify issues that are frightening or anxiety-provoking;
- thinking 'out loud' comments to encourage reflection on an issue or state of mind;
- reflective comments that recall themes or preoccupations;
- worker-related comments to encourage participants to challenge or confront the leader.

These interpretations are always purposeful—that is, they are aimed at moving the group forwards towards the achievement of its purpose. The extent to which these interpretations are 'good' interpretations will be able to be judged by the extent to which the group does move forward. Interpretations will, of course, differ considerably depending on the stage or phase of the group's life and development (see Chapter 8)—for example, whether it is the first or the last meeting. Again, the kind of group it is and the purpose it was set up to achieve (both of which are strongly influenced by the theoretical base which underpins its design and content) will result in differences in the nature and scope of the worker's interpretive acts.

How does the group worker make interpretations?

Here are some suggestions:

- When speaking in the group, it is wise to do so tentatively rather than categorically. It is always possible that the worker's interpretations will not be correct. For this reason, most group workers

phrase their comments and questions in such a way that participants can be engaged in exploring whether or not they make sense
to them. Tentative comments or questions give participants leeway
in how they might make use (or not) of the group worker's words
for themselves.

- The choice of words by the worker is important. Interpretations
can take the form of open-ended questions or of thoughts-in-
progress. It is good practice to adopt and use the words or metaphors
that participants themselves use, not only as a way of recognising
participants' contributions but also as a means of developing the
group's own particular language and culture. This is a practical way
of helping to establish and maintain the group's sense of identity.

- The interpretations the group worker makes are, as we discussed
earlier, derived from his/her participating and observing, listening,
remembering and thinking about this particular group-as-a-
whole that he/she is working with. It makes sense, then, that the
interpretations should, for the most part, be directed primarily
towards the group-as-a-whole, not individual participants. Often,
of course, the group worker will address an individual participant
but the interpretation made will be designed to facilitate the connections between that individual and other participants.

Contextualising: Working with diversity

The capacity to 'think group' brings with it an openness to the variety
and possibility within a collectivity. It presupposes a recognition of the
contextualised nature of knowing and understanding, for the group
occurs within a context that is not only constructed in the immediacy
of the physical surroundings but derives its particular meaning
from the social, economic and political–historical period in which it
is occurring. The questions 'What kind of a group is this? What is

happening here? What does this mean?' are answerable within our knowledge of the context.

The kinds of groups that are being established and the kinds of issues collective work addresses refer directly to the nature of the particular society in which the group exists (see Burkhardt 1982). For example, at the start of the twenty-first century, many Western liberal democracies are seeing increasing diversity amongst citizens. These demographic and political changes have immediate consequences for group workers. On a very practical level, group leaders need to ensure that they come to the task with capacities to work sensitively and effectively with the diverse experiences and situations of group participants. This requires a degree of self-awareness, given that our prejudices are often unconscious.

Recognising the limitations inherent in one's own (often unconscious) prejudices requires us to carefully review our own actions and reactions to the 'otherness' of others, and the likelihood that the group-as-a-whole may be subject to similar constraints. For example, with members from different ethnic communities in the group, the worker must have an openness to hearing them talk about their experience from their own perspective, avoiding taking for granted what he or she, as the leader, may assume will be their point of view. Where group members come from marginalised and minority groups, the worker requires skills in challenging prejudices and stereotyping and, at times, advocating on their behalf. The group leader requires skills that enable him/her to focus on helping members to gain more control over their lives, to become aware of and make use of their personal resources and to receive the support, where necessary, to confront situations where they experience inequality or oppression (Sachs 1991; Mullender and Ward 1991; Staub-Bernasconi 1991; Vinik and Levin 1991; Brown and Dickey 1992; Spence and Goldstein 1995; Butler and Wintram 1995; Toseland and Rivas 1998; Benjamin et al. 1997; Quinn 2000).

Staub-Bernasconi (1991, p. 80) points out, in relation to empowerment-oriented group work, that the group may provide a more egalitarian setting for participants than does a one-to-one relationship. In the group, members discover both their commonalities and their differences, and this may enable critical insights into their situation to emerge in ways which increase the power both of the individual and the group. 'Think group' thus also means 'think group-in-context', recognising the 'legitimate social differences and genuine similarities between races, classes, and sexes' (Burkhardt 1982, pp. 134–35). It is a stance which enables the group worker to attend simultaneously to two intersecting streams of information (see Flaherty 1999, p. 141): information from the external environment—what we know about social reality in this time and place; and information from the internal environment—our self-consciousness, cognitions and emotions. In 'thinking group' the group worker oscillates between the two, observing and participating in the interplay of objectivity and subjectivity.

In short, contextualising group work practice means that the group worker acts strategically to:

- recognise and acknowledge the diverse circumstances of group participants;
- identify differences as well as commonalities;
- provide space in the group for participants to talk about their commonalities and differences;
- avoid making assumptions about the circumstances of participants from oppressed or minority groups;
- where appropriate, take opportunities to advocate for participants from oppressed or minority groups;
- maintain a focus on the group-as-a-whole, being aware of the likelihood that prejudice may inhere at an unconscious level within the group-as-a-whole. In light of this, it is important to take opportunities when they arise to bring to consciousness those unconscious elements so that they can be worked with within the group-as-a-whole.

Summary

'Thinking group' refers to the conceptual frame from within which group workers approaches their practice in the group. However, to 'translate' this frame into actual strategies for working in the group requires that group workers develop their capacity to participate and observe, listen, remember, think, speak and attend to contextual factors impacting on group participants and on the group-as-a-whole.

7

FORMING A GROUP:
'The people in it create it'

In Chapter 2 we discussed the centrality of purpose. That was followed in Chapters 3, 4, 5 and 6 with a discussion of the relationship between purpose and theory and the nature and type of leadership characterising the group. These three elements—purpose, theory and leadership—are united in decisions made about what form the group is to take and who will comprise its membership. The key issues relevant to a discussion about forming a group are:

- group type; and
- group structure.

Before embarking on an exploration of these issues, however, it is important to recognise that making a decision about what kind of group to form is very much in the realm of the hypothetical: groups do not exist apart from, nor are they constituted except by, the individuals who begin working collectively together. Helen comments: 'What makes setting up a group really difficult [is] because you're doing it blind . . . you've got an idea for the group but you haven't got the people.'

In thinking about group type and structure, the leader or originator of the group is considering how best to release the creative and dynamic potential which several individuals can contribute to the service of a common purpose. Out of this collective coming together emerges the processes and dynamics of the group—the elements which leaders and participants work with over the life of the group. Thus decisions about group type and structure are decisions about group process. Type and structure reflect ways of organising and containing these emerging dynamics so that the group's purpose can be achieved.

forming a group

I just wanted to drop you all a note and let you know that I arrived safe and sound into Dulles Airport tonight at about 6.00 Thursday September 20 [nine days after the September 11, 2001 terrorist attacks by hijacked aircraft in New York and Washington]. It was an interesting flight. The airport in Denver was almost spooky, it was so empty and quiet. No one was in the line for the security check point when I got there so that went fairly smoothly, just x-ray of my bags and then a chemical test to be sure nothing explosive was on them. Then I waited two hours to board the plane. What happened after we boarded was interesting and I thought I would share it with you.

The pilot/captain came on the loudspeaker after the doors were closed. His speech went like this: 'First I want to thank you for being brave enough to fly today. The doors are now closed and we have no help from the outside for any problems that might occur inside this plane. As you could tell when you checked in, the government has made some changes to increase security in the airports. They have not, however, made any rules about what happens after those doors close. Until they do that, we have made our own rules and I want to share them with you.

'Once those doors closed, we only have each other. The security has taken care of a threat like guns with all of the increased scanning, etc. Then we have the supposed bomb. If you have a bomb, there is no need to tell me about it, or anyone else on this plane; you are already in control. So, for this flight, there are no bombs that exist on this plane. Now, the threats that are left are things like plastics, wood, knives, and other weapons that can be made or things like that which can be used as weapons. Here is our plan and our rules. If someone or several people stand up and say they are hijacking this plane, I want you all to stand up together. Then take whatever you have available to you and throw it at them. Throw it at their faces and heads so they will have to raise their hands to protect themselves. The very best protection you have against knives are the pillows and blankets. Whoever is close to these people should then try to get a blanket over their heads, then they won't be able to see. Once that is done, get them down and keep them there. Do not let them up. I will then land the plane at the closest airport and we WILL take care of them. After all, there are usually only a few of them and we are 200+ strong! We will not allow them to take over this plane. I find it interesting that the US Constitution begins with the words "We, the people"—that's who we are—THE people, and we will not be defeated.'

With that, the passengers on the plane all began to applaud, people had tears in their eyes, and we began the trip toward the runway. The flight attendant then began the safety speech. One of the things she said is that we are all so busy and live our lives at such a fast pace. She asked that everyone turn to their neighbours on either side and introduce themselves, tell each other something about your families and children, show pictures, whatever. She said: 'For today, we consider you family. We will treat you as such and ask that you do the same with us.'

During the flight we learned that, for the crew, this was their first flight since Tuesday's tragedies. It was a day that everyone leaned on each other and together everyone was stronger than any one person alone. It was quite an experience. You can imagine the feeling when that plane touched down at Dulles and we heard: 'Welcome to Washington Dulles Airport, where the local time is 5.40.' Again, the cabin was filled with applause. (original author unknown)

This example demonstrates very poignantly how a collection of people can be formed into a group under potentially threatening circumstances. What is particularly noteworthy here is the role of the pilot and cabin crew in creating (through their words) a sense of solidarity, empowerment and community among disparate people who had similar knowledge and anxieties but as yet were strangers to each other.

In forming a group, leaders are working on the basis of hunches— or, better still, decisions informed by knowledge and experience ('practice wisdom') about what structures, when set in place, will effect the kinds of processes that will emerge. In the above example, for instance, we can see the ways in which the pilot and cabin crew facilitated the development of common bonds, beginning trust and a sense of shared power in dealing with adversity.

In Douglas's view (1993), the group is a resource system and in creating it, the group worker's task is to develop members' access to as many resources (such things as knowledge, power, experience, networks) as possible. The kinds of resources which become available for members to access will be determined by decisions made at the outset, which are designed to focus the group's energy on achieving its purpose. These decisions may refer to such things as who will be in the group, who will be excluded, the number of group meetings, the frequency of meetings, and so on. For example, a decision to limit a group to women with recurrent breast cancer is made in order to facilitate a focus on the experience of that disease and to build supportive emotional linkages from this basis amongst participants who share that disease in common. When men with the same diagnosis are not included, this may indicate an assumption that gender is relevant to building a particular kind of relationship which is predicated on a sense of gender identity held in common.

Again, a decision to limit the number of group meetings to, for example, six weekly sessions of two hours, as in Robyn's group, indicates that the group's purpose—in this case, learning about and sharing experiences of parenting step-children—can be achieved within that time. It also means that other possibilities, such as an in-depth exploration of the psychological impact of step-parenting, will not be pursued. By way of contrast, Bernard's psychoanalytic group meets five days per week for one hour and participants attend for years rather than months. Its purpose is to achieve insight, which takes time: 'You get to know people in a narrow context but it's a very deep context . . . it really is very intensive. I think if you're going to do it it's a benefit to do it [as often as this].'

In summary, the decision about group form derives from purpose and theory. It is a decision which recognises the uncertainty of the enterprise but puts in place structures which are designed to enable the purpose to be achieved in the best possible way. While there are no hard and fast rules about the formation and structuring of groups, most group workers draw on accumulated theoretical and practice knowledge, research findings and their own experience to determine guidelines under which their group will function.

Ethics

The decision to form a group is always accompanied by a recognition of the possible ethical implications of doing so. The type of group proposed and the form it will take will vary depending on the situation and condition of those for whom the group is intended. In the human services, many groups target vulnerable populations—those who may belong to marginal or minority communities, people experiencing life crises, people struggling with everyday problems in living.

Ethical considerations underpin all social practices and interventions, and group work is no exception. Practitioners emphasise the two primary ethical principles of informed consent and minimising harm. In the context of the group, this means ensuring that potential and actual participants are aware of the purpose of the group and the likely activities and processes involved before they agree or consent to join. Where participants do not volunteer to join—for example, when they are mandated to attend—they require clear explanations of what will be expected of them with regard to attendance and participation. For example, many of the participants in Chris's group for men who are violent are referred from the child protection or criminal justice systems. While acknowledging that none of them wishes to be there, Chris also recognises that the group symbolises hope: '[there is an] alternative to violence, there really is a choice . . . there's an opportunity here . . .' His pre-group assessment interviews are an important ethical component in enabling potential participants 'to identify that they have to change their behaviour'—in other words, to make them aware that the purpose of the group is to achieve behavioural change and potential participants enter it with this knowledge.

It is the responsibility of the group leader to ensure that participants are not damaged by their participation. This means that, in the first instance, confidentiality must be assured. Participants are usually informed that what is discussed within the group remains exclusively with that group. Of course, in some situations this will be a limited confidentiality. Should members disclose illegal activities or behaviour that threatens the life or well-being of themselves or someone else, action may be taken to involve outside authorities. Potential participants need to be made aware of such arrangements before they join the group if taking action of this kind is within the group worker's mandate (Schoener and Luepker 1996).

Other ethical considerations designed to protect group members from harm may include proscribing attendance if someone is affected by drugs or alcohol. For example, Bridget's group—the Women's Circus—requires participants to do physical performance, so safety (both physical and emotional) is very important. Users of drugs or alcohol are only excluded if they are adversely affected at the time of rehearsals. She comments:

With new members in particular [we're] big on physical and psychological safety. We make sure that there's a circle at the end of each workshop and everyone's got a chance to talk about how it's been for them. The trainer talks through some of the things women might experience if they're using their bodies in different ways that bring up emotional stuff... [we also] reinforce basic safety rules—like you don't do anything that's too much for you ... how to be involved safely in an empowering way...

Groups can be emotional hothouses and the group leader has a vital responsibility to ensure that members are adequately protected from one another and from the leader (see Schoener and Luepker 1996). This requires the leader to be alert to, and capable of, containing emotion within the group in ways that can be constructive and productive for all. Janet, in her focus group work, noted that she as leader required skills in balancing individual vulnerabilities with the purposes of the research and the group dynamics. She comments: 'One of the consumers was very disturbed by his experience so he took over—it was very hard to contain him in the group.' Chris's group for men who are violent made similar demands on him as leader:

I'm very clear about where I stand with the stuff and I'm clear about the parameters—the balance between them being individuals, but in terms of the group atmosphere having boundaries ... they need to be secure that what's said here stays here, that they're not getting beaten up by someone they challenged, that when they disclose really hard stuff, it's not going to be treated like shit.

They're going to be listened to respectfully . . . and heard. That does happen I think and gives them confidence [to participate].

The group leader's ethical responsibility to the group suggests that his/her own agenda and behaviour must be constantly under scrutiny (see Schoener and Luepker 1996). A study by Yalom and Lieberman (1974) into 'casualties' in encounter groups—those who endured a significant negative outcome which was caused by their participation in the group—identified a particular leadership style as a causal factor. Such a leadership style was characterised by high stimulus input, aggression, charisma, support, intrusiveness, and individual as opposed to interpersonal or group focus for interventions. It had particularly negative consequences for vulnerable individuals—those with a low self-concept and unrealistically high expectations and anticipations of change. These damaging outcomes for some participants highlight the importance of group workers seeking peer or individual supervision and ensuring that their work is subject to constant self-reflection and critique.

Types Of group

In thinking about the form of group to be established it is useful to review existing ways of categorising different group types. Groups have been classified in a number of ways in order to distinguish their different purposes and characteristics. How one classifies them is, of course, open to debate. Given, as we noted in Chapter 3, that similar groups can emerge from different theoretical orientations, theory is not a useful basis for classification. However, there are two ways in which, broadly speaking, groups can be classified: by type and by content.

In an important and influential paper in 1966 (see Papell 1997), Papell and Rothman outlined three models of social work with groups. These models affirm the relationship between group work and the social context in which it is practised. The type of group formed invariably reflects the different emphases characterising different eras in the history of the development of the social work profession and thus changes in the 'wider' social and historical context in which group work is embedded (see Burkhardt 1982). The *social goals model*, sharing ground with notions of the group as power base (see Chapter 3), grew out of group work in the settlement houses and community centres in the early years of the twentieth century. The focus was upon the group as a demonstration of commitment to democratic principles of participation and collective action to achieve social change. The *remedial model*, sharing ground with notions of the group as comprising individuals and containing properties (see Chapter 3), emerged during the 1950s and took a treatment-oriented approach to group work. The group was conceptualised and used as an intervention strategy in parallel with case work and community work. The *reciprocal model* or *mutual aid group*, sharing ground with notions of the group as a system (see Chapter 3), emerged in the latter half of the last century, placing attention on working with the relationships amongst members and their connections with the social environment in which the group was embedded.

Shulman's work (1999, p. 327) differs from Papell and Rothman's (see Papell 1997) in proposing a content specific typology of groups. His typology is useful in that it is broad enough to incorporate a range of different kinds of groups while categorising them in specific terms in relation to their central features. Shulman notes four types:

- *Support and rehabilitation groups:* these are suited to those who are experiencing life crises such as divorce, a serious illness or the death of someone close. The purpose of support and rehabilitation groups is to generate support within the group to assist individuals to manage the stress in their lives. Self-help as well as various kinds of mutual aid groups may be assigned to this category. The Breast Cancer Therapy Group is a good example of this type of group.

- *Growth and education groups:* these groups are designed for people who are encountering major life developmental challenges, such as entering parenthood or adolescence. They may be relevant to people whose developmental progress has been delayed or inhibited by, for example, the onset of a mental illness. The purpose of growth and education groups is for participants to learn relevant competencies and skills so that they can achieve various developmental tasks, such as managing independent community living or strengthening parental capacities. Psycho-educational and self-help groups may belong to this category. Robyn's step-parenting group is a good example of a growth and education group, as is Heather's 'socio-educational' group for women.

- *Task and action groups:* these are characteristic of social action and community development groups and committees. Their primary purpose is to accomplish tasks rather than focus on generating support for individuals or assisting them to accomplish developmental tasks. Social action groups, committees and advocacy groups may belong to this category. Helen's social action group and Maria's self-help and advocacy group addressing fertility issues are good examples of these types of groups. The Women's Circus which Bridget belongs to also reflects some similar characteristics.

- *Recapitulation and restitution groups:* these are groups which focus on the development of an individual's insight into the nature and meaning of their behaviour and life experiences. The purpose of recapitulation and restitution groups is to review life events and explore unconscious and conscious material and analyse it in order to strengthen individuals' cognitive, emotional and intellectual self-understanding. Psychotherapeutic and counselling groups may belong to this category. Bernard's psychoanalytically oriented psychotherapy group and Cynthia's support and therapy group for mothers with terminal illness and their children are examples of recapitulation and restitution groups.

Classifying groups according to these kinds of typology alerts us to the importance of different purposes and their different consequences with regard to the kinds of processes and dynamics which different types of groups are designed to achieve. However, where groups are classified according to *content*, process assumes less importance in relation to the need to have detailed knowledge about the specific characteristics and attributes of particular populations. For example, we might review what is known about the needs of adolescents—in social, cultural, educational, physical and emotional terms—before a particular kind of group is designed to achieve positive outcomes directly referring to aspects of the way adolescents' needs are interpreted. A focus on *content* rather than *process* suggests that the group worker will have very specialised knowledge about the particular needs of this particular group. However, to that must be added an understanding of the processes and dynamics of groups if workers are to ensure that the group is formed, developed and sustained to the best possible effect for participants (see Papell 1997). A focus on *content* alone can be problematic. It is the interchange, communication and dialogue occurring amongst members which create the group. This is at the centre of the leader's attention. How to understand, work with and shape this process distinguishes the practice of group work from, for example, working with individuals in a group.

Structure

When the term 'structure' is used in relation to groups, it refers to the establishment of boundaries within which the work of the group takes place. By boundaries I am referring to those elements which separate the group as a bounded social entity from other aspects of everyday social life. By establishing a boundary—a group—we are determining what is inside and what is outside the group; who is inside and who is outside; what belongs to the group and what is separate from it. The sense of boundary and how it is to be defined for a particular group

117

clearly have a significant impact on the kinds of relationships that will develop within the group, the relationship the group will have with the outside world, and how these boundaries will impact on sustaining or inhibiting relationships within the group. Perhaps most importantly of all, boundaries serve to set the conditions for the development of a sense of group identity and to influence the degree of cohesion experienced by members (see Petronio et al. 1998). The fact that an entity is perceived as a group at all is determined by the existence of boundaries. In turn, knowledge of these boundaries prefigures our response to it. For example, if we know that this is a group for carers of people with HIV/AIDS, our response to it—our expectations of what it will be like and of who will be in it—will influence our reaction to it well before we encounter the group.

So, in considering how to structure a group, we are deciding what boundaries to establish. While these boundaries are strongly determined by purpose and theory, we can explore in greater detail some of the elements which operate to structure a group and determine the nature of the processes which may emerge. We will consider six structures:

- decision-making, rules and guidelines;
- time;
- open or closed format;
- size;
- membership;
- activities.

Decision-making

Groups can be thought of as the embodiment of a structure for decision-making. This will be evident in whether or not the group has a hierarchical structure with a designated leader and designated members, or whether it is structured as a collective with a flat and moveable leadership structure in which every member has an equal responsibility to take charge of the group on various occasions to achieve various ends. Or decision-making might begin with the leader and evolve to the members. What happens will depend on purpose.

Rules or guidelines for how work is to be done in the group, and by whom, may be established at the outset. For example, in an ongoing group, the leader's role may be to assess potential members and to introduce them at various times when the leader believes this is appropriate. Leaders might also instigate rules about attendance, or emphasise the importance of 'taking turns' in talking, or of members sharing various pieces of information with the group—for example, about any crises or life-changing decisions they are taking. Where participants have particular characteristics—for example people living with psychiatric disabilities—the group may be characterised by flexibility and 'permission' for participants to come and go as necessary.

Members themselves might introduce other rules or norms about what they expect of one another—for example, to come on time, not to use physical force, to give one another space to talk, to listen to the leader, and so on. The decision-making structure adopted and the rules or guidelines determined, play a part in establishing power relations in a group. Thus power relationships *do* structure the group, although often in quite subtle ways. They are important elements to recognise and understand in order to shape them towards constructive ends which serve to maximise the participatory and democratic potential inherent in collective work.

Time

The duration of the group's existence and the length and frequency of meetings form definite boundaries which specify how much time is available for the group to work and, as a consequence, what it is possible to achieve. For example, a long-term group such as a psycho-analytically oriented psychotherapy group may never end—as long as the leaders remain committed to it. Other groups—for example, single-session groups (Ebenstein 1998)—have a considerably shortened period of time to achieve their purpose. Groups which meet for a specified number of sessions—usually between eight and twelve (Magen 1995)—often rely on a carefully designed program of activities which will sustain them over that period, and evidence a clear rationale for the inclusion of material for exploration over that time span. Groups may meet daily or weekly, or less frequently, depending upon their purpose. The more frequently the group meets, the more intensive that group experience is likely to be. The time structure may also be flexible—for example, the group may convene for a number of meetings held in close succession and then move to weekly or monthly meetings. Such structure may be relevant when participants have experienced a trauma, such as a cyclone or the unexpected death of a colleague. Immediate work to manage the emotional impact may then move into a longer-term working-through of the issues.

The length of meetings usually ranges from one to two hours, but some task and action groups may set longer meeting times as their purpose is to achieve a particular targeted outcome rather than to engage in emotionally demanding exchanges between members. For the latter purpose, a shorter time-frame may be useful in containing emotion and preventing the 'over-exposure' of vulnerable participants. Thus the boundaries set by time clearly affect group processes (what happens in the group) and the kinds of phases which characterise the life of the group, such as beginnings, middles and ends. These will be discussed in the next chapter.

Open and closed groups

Whether or not a group will be designed to exist over a predetermined period of time with predetermined activities and a fixed membership is clearly a boundary decision.

An *open* group is one which, by definition, is ongoing. Members join and leave when it is appropriate and the group activity will reflect this. Thus an open group is unlikely to have a set format but rather will rely on the agenda brought by different members which fits with the overall purpose of the group. An example of this kind of open group is a therapy group such as the one Bernard belonged to: 'We all just go in and sit down and anybody can say anything they like—there isn't a sense of time being divided among members of the group.'

A *closed* group, on the other hand, follows a particular program. Growth and education groups, which include psychoeducation groups, are a good example of this type of closed group. In such groups, a program of information, didactic input, videos and role-plays focused around a particular issue, are offered along with opportunities for discussion and learning. Membership is generally closed—that is, new members are not admitted once the program has commenced. Professional development groups and psychoeducational groups frequently are structured along these lines (see also the example of the Parenting in Recovery Program in Chapter 3).

The combination of an open and a closed structure can also be relevant to achieving a group's purpose. Such a structure would characterise a program in which participants entered a closed time-limited group and then progressed to an ongoing open group. This may be appropriate where the purpose was to address the needs of people with particular problems who could benefit from educational material delivered in a focused way and then move on to explore that in the context of their lives and the ongoing stresses they encounter. Participants might also move in the opposite direction—beginning in the open group and moving into the closed. Thus the open group may have members entering, leaving and re-entering at different points, but all will have participated in, or will be about to participate in, the closed group. This combined arrangement may allow agencies to offer a continuous program with flexibility and the potential to respond to a need for immediate group participation if that should arise.

Heather's women's support and discussion group, which she describes as a 'socio-educational group', demonstrates a combined open and closed structure with opportunities for participants to be involved in the selection of topics. These have included 'decision-making, goal-setting, becoming and staying motivated, guilt, dealing with dominating behaviour, stories and poems that have touched us, dealing with the news [on TV], dealing with conflict'. Heather comments on the group's structure:

> The initial six week part remains very open and women frequently join several weeks into the program. Our decision to allow this is quite deliberate and reflects our experience that women's lives don't always go according to plan and that some women may take several attempts to actually make it to the group. The membership of the ongoing monthly group is limited to those women who have attended the initial six-week program (or at least some weeks of it) so this, in a sense, is closed except for two new intakes of members each year. (written communication)

A decision to form an open or a closed group will be taken after considering both the group's purpose and the characteristics of potential participants. Different kinds of skills will be required of the leader. For example, a closed group may be appropriate where participants require stability and a sense of safety if, for instance, they have experienced abuse or domestic violence (Roxburgh and DVIRC 1994; Shaw et al. 1999). An open group may be more appropriate where participants are working on issues shared in common but which have different significance for individuals—for example, chronic or terminal illness. Where the purpose of the group is to assist people in confronting anxiety-provoking and existential issues (such as life and death, pain, coping with chronic illness) an open group may allow support to develop and be maintained even as the membership changes through illness or the death of participants (Spiegel and Spira 1991).

Where the leader is working with a closed group, this may require that he/she takes a more dominant role in influencing the pace of work and is more directive in ensuring that the group's purposes are achieved by the conclusion of the group (Sunderland 1997/98). The leader of an open group may, in contrast, take a less directive role and allow group members greater influence in shaping the group.

Size

The number of participants in a group is a significant issue for consideration. Too few participants—three or less—may intensify relationships in ways which, depending on the reason members are in the group, could be experienced as inhibiting participation by over-exposing individual vulnerabilities. Fewer people also reduce the number of different personalities, minds and experiences the group can draw upon. The power of the leader may be experienced as particularly threatening in very small groups—and even more so if there are two leaders.

On the other hand, a group that is very large—more than twelve members—may limit opportunities to participate in the time available. The chance that smaller sub-groupings or factions will develop is increased. Sub-groups can fracture the cohesiveness of the collectivity and may lead to competitive behaviour which distracts the group from achieving its purpose. However, very large groups, such as Lou's positive ageing group, are designed to be so, having 80–100 members. She reflects:

To some extent the individual experience gets lost but is also magnified in the setting . . . in a room of 80 your voice can be heard and you can do so much inner work but at the same time you're anonymous within that setting. [This is] almost a contradictory or counter-intuitive perspective on it but it happens . . . it's really lovely, these people losing themselves in a crowd only to find themselves in a crowd.

(For an exploration of some of the psychodynamics of large groups, see Main 1989.)

Practice, wisdom and experience suggest that the most satisfactory number of participants in support and rehabilitation, and recapitulation and restitution groups is between seven and ten members. This number provides sufficient space for participants to be heard, to be listened to, to find support and challenge, and to achieve a diverse range of purposes. It is also a size which is within the capacity of the leader(s) to attend to the processes, dialogue and exchange taking place without being overwhelmed. Growth and education and task and action groups can work with larger numbers, perhaps up to fifteen or twenty. In task and action groups, a smaller core of four to six members usually takes responsibility for the work of the group.

Membership

It's not just a matter of you bringing a group of people together and various things happen—the sorts of people you bring together can change the sort of group you have . . . (Helen)

Leaders talk about recruiting or selecting members; participants talk about joining a group. This difference in language tells us much about the initial difference in perspectives of leaders and (potential) participants. How both parties find a point of connection whereby their own agenda, expectations and anticipations can jointly be met through their participation in the group may occur through pre-group interviews or, in the case of a task and action group, participants may self-select. In both cases, it may take time and experience in the group to determine whether or not the group provides the kind of process desired and of use to the participant.

Many group workers firmly hold to the need to assess potential members' suitability for a group. In this process, individuals are to an extent being redefined as potential group members (Douglas 1993). The purpose of pre-group interviews is to attempt to discover some of the following:

- the willingness of potential participants to join the group. If they are mandated to do so, to what extent will this element of coercion interfere with their capacity to benefit from the group?
- the nature of the problem or issue the potential participant has and how this can be met through the group;
- the potential participant's suitability for a group—that is, their ability to become confortable in talking and working with others and, depending upon the group's purpose, their capacity to deal with emotional vulnerability;
- the likelihood that the potential participant's personality will blend with others in the group;
- their willingness to commit the time and energy required to be a consistent group member;
- the potential participant's intellectual and cognitive capacities that will allow them to benefit from the group;
- the potential participant's physical and/or sensory capacities—for example, ability, mobility, hearing, sight—which will enable them to contribute to the group's program or activities;
- the potential participant's emotional or mental state and the extent to which the group is able to accommodate fluctuations and changes in the person's capacity to participate;
- the potential participant's cultural or ethnic background and the extent to which the group is designed to accommodate diversity;
- the language skills of the potential participant;
- the potential participant's age and personal circumstances, such as marital status and sexuality and the extent to which the group is designed to accommodate diversity;
- the potential participant's situation with regard to finances, transport, employment and child care which may determine their availability to attend the group.

This checklist is not exhaustive and its relevance lies in assisting both leader and potential participant to gauge whether or not this particular group and its purpose will fit with the individual's needs. Helen comments: 'You have to be really clear who is in the group and what's an appropriate structure and process, not just for the goal but for the people.'

Brown (1989, pp. 27–51; see also Bloch and Aveline 1996) proposes several principles which underlie group leaders' decisions about group membership. These concern homogeneity, heterogeneity, balance and compatibility.

Homogeneity—the elements which members have in common— is important for cohesion. Members of the Breast Cancer Therapy Group commented:

> We can speak quite honestly about our disease whereas most of us would agree that outside of the group we protect our families and other friends . . . the main link we have is our breast cancer and all the stuff that happens to us—issues like hair loss, body image, wellness . . .

Heterogeneity refers to those elements which members do not share but which allow the possibility for challenge and for change. Bridget notes:

> You don't have to be a particular type of woman to join except in so far as committing to the aims . . . it's the aims which unite and one of the aims is diversity in terms of fitness and shape and size—it's not the sort of group you go to to be with women like yourself.

Janet concurs in relation to her focus group work:

> Focus groups are good because you make an environment where people can have different points of view and it's OK—you develop these different points of view . . .

Balance refers to the extent to which members are not too distant from one another in terms of age or ethnicity or social class, so that common ground can be found. Where this is ignored, the consequences are problematic. Bernard notes:

The age thing can be a bit of a problem. A 23-year-old woman had a bit of difficulty in relating to the group with the gender differences (nine men and one woman) and the age differences (40+ years) . . . she didn't stay long . . .

Compatibility refers to the extent to which each individual's needs complement those of at least one other person—for example, at least two people may be struggling with feelings of loneliness or inadequacy with regard to their social relationships. Anecdotally, some group leaders refer to this as the 'Noah's Ark' principle: an issue or problem should always be shared by a minimum of two people.

We noted earlier in this section that many group workers prefer to offer pre-group assessment interviews, both to enable them to ascertain an individual's suitability for the group and for the potential participant to decide whether or not the group might meet their needs and expectations. However, not all group workers believe that this is a necessary first step. Some argue that a pre-group interview places the group worker in a pre-eminently powerful position, both in their own estimation and in that of the potential participant. The pre-group interview may be interpreted as an assertion that the group worker is an expert who can predict the outcome for an individual and for the group. Heather, for example, in her women's support and discussion group, believes that women have a capacity to be self-monitoring. Instead of pre-group assessment interviews, she prefers to 'be open to what the women bring themselves and letting that happen'.

In task and action groups—especially those with a social action orientation—the emphasis is likely to be on people joining the group rather than being recruited. It is the issue or problem that brings people to the group, often independently of any intermediary. Maria comments in relation to her self-help and advocacy group: 'anyone can join. I want the whole world!' Similarly, Helen's social action group concerned 'an issue (which) was very clear cut and something people felt strongly about . . . it was very much a group for a purpose and it brought people together—some quite disparate people—it worked well for what it did . . .'

Gender

While we have already noted some of the issues relevant to the gender of leaders in Chapter 4, decisions about the gender composition of groups are again key boundary issues which structure the kinds of group processes likely to emerge. The purposes driving the establishment of the group are of course central to this decision. Weeks (1988; see also Reed and Garvin 1983, 1996; Butler and Wintram 1995; Bernardez 1996), for example, details the benefits which women working together collectively can achieve. These include such things as enabling women to bring social and political perspectives into their lives, assisting women to make sense of their experiences, assisting them to explore their relationships with other women, and enabling women to define, interpret and name their experiences without seeking male support or validation.

Wright and Gould (1996, p. 342) note that gender composition impacts significantly on both the quality and the content of the inter-action that occurs in the group. In single-gender groups, participants are not confronted with the 'other'; rather, they have the opportunity to work with one another in a very direct way provided that the poten-tial for collusion to occur is recognised and addressed. Bob comments in relation to his pro-feminist all-male group:

> We struggle to find ways of connecting with each other as men
> that are not at the expense of women, and most forms of male

bonding are at the expense of women . . . we endeavour to find ways of connecting with each other as men that do involve intimacy and sharing and self-disclosure but are not based on creating the 'otherness' of women . . .

Heather, who co-leads a women-only support and discussion group, makes a similar point:

It's like it doesn't have to be the ideal of what is female—it could be anything—but as soon as you put a man in a room then I know that I'm a woman and something else happens . . . and it's just about taking away all those social prescriptions that I think we inherit and experience. It's much more liberating for women [to be in a women-only group].

Groups which are homogenous in relation to gender can provide safety for participants to break away from gender stereotypes and take risks in their self-exploration. Heather argues:

I feel like the fact that men aren't there forces women to explore and be something else. If men are there they do dominate and take up a lot of group space and it's hard for women not to fall into subservient positions . . . there's just an automatic deferment by women . . . You want to give women the opportunity to find space to be whoever . . .

Groups which are heterogenous with regard to gender provide different opportunities for participants, particularly in relation to the exploration of interpersonal relationships between men and women. Depending on the purpose—for example, Robyn's psychoeducational step-parenting group, relationships between men and women may be an important focus. However, regardless of the group's purpose, gender composition—whether heterogenous or homogenous—

cannot but have a significant impact on the way members work together just as it does in wider society. How men and women make use of the group situation will differ. In fact, Schoenholtz-Reed (1996, p. 238) argues that: 'The mixed gender therapy group most clearly revives the social role expectations and tensions that present between the sexes in the culture' (see also Wright and Gould 1996). The consequences which flow from this—for example, in relation to men's and women's help-seeking behaviour, availability and willingness to participate in groups—are important to recognise in planning and forming groups (see Walsh 1994; Tudiver and Talbot 1999; Spink 2000).

Age

The age of group members is an important issue in deciding to form or join a group. Many groups are formed to accommodate people at particular points in the life cycle—childhood, adolescence, young adulthood, adulthood, late life. The assumption here is that people who share an age grouping are likely to have various things in common—for example, tastes in music, clothing, entertainment, or to be in the midst of various life cycle stage-related experiences, such as parenthood, retirement, entering the workforce, and so on. Corey (2000, pp. 164–73), drawing usefully on Erikson's stages of psycho-sexual development, argues that on a psychosocial level, individuals negotiate various emotional tasks from infancy to maturity. These have implications for how people may use the group processes, depending upon their age and the stage of psychosexual/psychosocial development they are encountering.

Thus particular issues or 'problems in living' will arise at different times in the life cycle, such as learning to live with loss which may characterise late life, or establishing a sense of purpose or identity which may challenge young adults, or learning how to trust and engage with others which may confront children and adolescents. Working with these particular kinds of issues is often seen as very effectively done in group settings. In the profession of youth work, for instance, working with groups is considered a core activity, given the age of their 'constituency' (see Benjamin et al. 1997, pp. 59–64).

Homogeneity in terms of age is often a priority in forming the group. For example, the workers in an ongoing psychotherapeutic group which has as its purpose working with adults who are depressed or finding difficulty in establishing and maintaining personal relationships are careful to select participants aged between 30 and 50 years. This age span allows for enough homogeneity in terms of age, heterogeneity in terms of specific life experiences, and overall compatibility in terms of the particular kinds of problems faced. The workers consider that anyone more than five years older or younger might unbalance the group and could mean that the group would not gel. It would also increase the likelihood that 'outliers' might face marginalisation and exclusion from the group majority.

Of course, these considerations regarding the age of participants are closely connected to the purpose of the group. Where groups are designed to achieve particular psychological, behavioural or social goals, homogeneity, heterogeneity, compatibility and balance are important criteria which may be relevant to the formation of the group and the selection of participants. Where the group has formed primarily in order to achieve a political or social change objective, age may have little bearing. In Helen's social action group, for example, participants from a wide range of backgrounds, political persuasions, nationalities, professions and trades combined forces—age was largely irrelevant.

Diversity

The diversity of ethnic and racial characteristics of group members will similarly have a significant impact on the way members work together. Thus, in forming a group, decisions about the extent to which racial and ethnic diversity will be accommodated require the worker to understand their likely impact on members and on the collective work of the group (Olarte 1996; Flannery et al. 2000). This means that the group worker must appreciate that group members may bring with them into the group the effects of minority status, of a history of racism and oppression which they may have been subject to, or an experience of stigma and discrimination. Other factors, such as differences in values, acceptable behaviours, language usage, the place and influence of family and other community members, must also be taken into account. Reviewing the literature on race discrimination in group work, Brown (1992) concludes from a British perspective that individuals are most comfortable in groups with those who are racially similar. He cautions against stereotyping or generalising about different ethnic groups and their preferred ways of working collectively—for example, whether an active or passive leadership style is preferred. However, he does identify that, amongst different ethnic groups, readiness to self-disclose, and to use politeness or confrontation, may vary. Brown (1992) concludes his review of the literature by suggesting that group work approaches which are culturally sensitive, concrete, actively led, environmentally focused and give attention to problem resolution are likely to be viewed positively by ethnic minority participants. Dowds (1996) provides an example of working with a group designed to promote sensitive inter-cultural understanding among patients with serious mental illness. He identifies (1996, p. 75) the principles of ethnic-sensitive group work practice which underpinned the group: a present-time focus, a structured activity with structured theme-focused discussion, active leadership and teamwork, cultural sharing and immersion in a culturally specific ritual, and respect for and empowerment of a particular cultural group. Annie Wu King (1988, pp. 80–81) offers a thought-provoking account of her group experience from the 'inside':

> Our attempts to escape from loneliness into relatedness have been researched and prescribed for in various ways. I remember an experience I had when I joined a T-group (sensitivity training

group) after living in Central Java, Indonesia, for more than four years. During the mini-marathon at the close of the six weeks of regular meetings, I recall how surprised I was then when someone [an American] told me that they had been upset with me because I was unwilling to share anything about myself. I realised then that I had absorbed more Javanese culture than I had been aware of. As I saw it, I had been quite open and willing to talk but was often 'cut off' by others with their busy agenda to 'get things out'. To the American I was somehow lacking assertiveness and openness; to the Javanese I was behaving appropriately. The facilitator of the group acknowledged that I had made him uncomfortable because I was physically disabled and he, therefore, found it difficult to address me and especially to confront me! Systematized relating had not allowed for individual differences.

Activities

The activities proposed for the group are the media through which the group's purpose will be met. As such, activities place a boundary around what is to occur within the group and indicate the choice the group leader has made about why these activities, in relation to all other possible activities, are the ones which will be offered. The physical location of the group will have some bearing on what kind of activities are possible—for example, the space available, other activities taking place in the building at the same time, accessibility for disabled people and children, and so on. For some groups, the physical arrangements of the room, the provision of particular kinds of furniture and decorations may be particularly important in demonstrating a recognition of cultural sensitivity towards what might create a welcoming and attractive environment—often the first and essential step in engaging participants in the process (see, for example, Links Project 1996). In addition, the type and range of activities will vary according to the group's purpose, the people in the group, the leaders' and members' creativity, the availability of resources and the suitability of the venue.

The age of group participants will influence the kinds of activities to be engaged in. For example, groups for children (such as Cynthia's) need to take into account the more limited verbal abilities of participants, which suggests that games or painting or work with clay might be more useful in helping the children communicate and express their concerns than talk-based work. Group work with adolescents and young adults has long been the particular focus of youth workers, especially with regard to team and outdoor activities as vehicles for establishing and strengthening their sense of identity and movement towards independence. Providing activities for groups of young people which can engage and challenge them at the same time as containing and tolerating rebellion and risk-taking might be especially demanding. (See Ivey et al. 2001 for some useful ideas in working with children and adolescents in groups.)

Some thought needs to be given to the physical demands that activities might require and the capacity of participants to do them safely and without anxiety. How the space in the room is to be used may be another decision to be made—for example, how close or distant participants are to be from one another, whether people will be seated on chairs in a circle, or cushions on the floor, and so on. If the group is to be technology-based with members meeting via the telephone or the internet (see Schopler et al. 1998; McGrath and Berdahl 1998), particular consideration will need to be given to how participants communicate and work with each other under these conditions.

Group activities may include 'nothing'—that is, only what members choose to talk about or be silent about in the group—to lectures, videos, painting, and so on. Activities reflect theoretical perspectives and knowledge about how individuals learn, about how insight is facilitated, and about how action leads to change. For example, in the psychoanalytic group, Bernard comments:

You'll do best in therapy if what you bring in are things about yourself that you don't understand or that to you seem irrational and that's why [the leader] encourages people to bring in dreams because they are your own creation and they give a clue to things about you . . .

Cynthia's group for children whose mothers are in palliative care or receiving cancer treatment works through 'the use of a "non-verbal toolbox"—a potpourri of artistic mediums'. Together the children and their mothers develop a workbook which records the feelings in the family about their impending loss. The child makes a gift which is given to the mother; it is 'the child's perception of what's important to mum . . . mum's favourite flower might be jasmine so we have jasmine as a liaising tool and then after mum's death the connection with mum is still intact, accessible . . .'

Chris's group for men who are violent begins with the circulation of an agreement sheet which details such things as the benefits and pitfalls of being in the group, where responsibility for behaviour lies, confidentiality, and so on. This is followed by the men telling their stories one by one whilst others comment or challenge. The leaders might extrapolate and draw from these contributions important issues or lessons for the men to consider with regard to their behaviour. Role-play and feedback might develop from this.

Helen's social action group engaged in various activities including establishing a picket line, holding a public meeting and informing the media—all of which were designed to draw attention to the issue raised and to pressure for change.

Summary

So far we have discussed those issues relevant to the formation of a group. Forming a group is the first step in transforming the group's purpose into a process through which it can be achieved. As we have noted, a number of decisions need to be made in order to carefully think through the relationship between the purpose the group is to have and the structure that is to be adopted. By way of summary, guidelines for making these decisions are noted on a checklist below. Of course, not all the issues identified here will be relevant to every group and the answer to one question may be relevant to several.

- What is the initial purpose this group is to serve?
- What is your theoretical framework—or how have you problematised this issue?
- Who is the group for?
- Who (at least initially) will lead the group? Will it be co-led? Why?
- Do you intend the leadership to change or evolve? If not, why not? If so, in what way and to whom?
- What ethical issues may arise in view of the likely group members and the group's purpose? How will these be managed, or in what way will the group be designed to accommodate them?
- Where will the group meetings be held? Why?
- What particular rules or guidelines may need to be put in place at the outset?
- Will the group be open or closed? A combination of both? Why?
- How often will the group meet? Why?
- Over what period of time? Why?
- How long will meetings be? Why?
- How many participants will initially be in the group? Why?
- Will participants:
  - be homogenous in terms of age, gender, ethnicity, etc.?
  - be heterogenous in terms of age, gender, ethnicity, etc.?
- How will participants be recruited? Will they volunteer?
- Will they be assessed before they are accepted? Why? Why not?

- What physical arrangements do you have in mind, e.g. people sitting in a circle, at tables, on the floor, etc.? Why?
- What activities are planned?
- What is the rationale for these activities?
- Are they to be sequenced? If so, why; if not, why not?
- What kind of a group process do you envisage will be created by the decisions you have made regarding group type and structure?
- Do you have to seek support or approval from the auspicing agency for this proposed group? What problems could you encounter? How will you deal with them?

8

THE LIFE OF THE GROUP:
'Laughter and tears'

I came to the group three years ago absolutely petrified of dying
... Over the time I've been coming I've slowly changed my
mind—a lot of fear has been removed. (Breast Cancer Therapy
Group)

There's more and more sharing as the weeks go on—much more
cross-fertilisation of ideas . . . (Robyn)

[The group is now] so different from what it was in the past . . .
(Maria)

These comments from group members and leaders describe well the
changes that participants notice over the duration of a group's life.
When people think about entering or forming a group, they may have
anxieties and fears about their acceptance or rejection by others, that
they will be unmasked in some way by exposing their vulnerabilities,
that they may lose their individuality and autonomy by being swept
along by forces they cannot control, that they may find themselves in

conflict with others which will damage them. Simultaneously, they may feel hopeful and excited at the possibility of gaining help or support from others, or that they may become a part of something that makes a difference in the world. These and many other thoughts, feelings, beliefs and assumptions are brought to the group by each individual participant. What happens over time to these ambivalent and sometimes contradictory emotions and thoughts is what makes up the life of the group. It is not possible to predict precisely what effect the experience of being in the group will have on individual emotions, thoughts and action, but we do know that they will be changed in some way. The group leader's task is to work to ensure that what happens can be shaped towards achieving the group's purpose. The materials the leader has at hand for doing this are the resources he/she brings, the resources group participants bring and the time-frame within which the group works. We can begin this discussion by exploring the notion of time as it refers to group work.

Time and the group

To think of the group as having a life is to think of it as a living thing, sharing a central characteristic of all animate and inanimate things— that is, of it existing within time and exhibiting the effects of time, namely change. Indeed, one of the best ways humans judge that time has elapsed is by noting that things are different, that what was present is no more or that something which was previously absent is now existing. Or it may be that we, as observers and participants, have changed to the extent that we notice different things at different times and interpret these varying observations as indicative of the passage of time. We may implicate time in creating these differences, or we may argue that we have altered our focus or interpreted the objects of our gaze differently from previously. A group is an enormously complex phenomenon which, once set in motion, may evolve, change, integrate and disintegrate in intricate and ever more varied and elaborate ways.

Being part of a group means that one is participating in a social and temporal process. Groups occur within an historical context characterised by the particular political, social and economic conditions operating in that context. This means that the group is a social structure which shares in and reflects the nature of the particular society in which it occurs. This is clearly obvious in social action and community development groups which are set up precisely in response to social and political conditions, with an agenda designed to influence those conditions in some way—for example, anti-globalisation groups active at various World Economic Forum meetings. It is less obviously the case with other groups such as support and rehabilitation, recapitulation and restitution, or growth and education groups, which seem to place their focus on the more immediate problems of living that people face. However, the nature of economic and political life at any given historical period will be impacting on human action whether or not individuals are aware of it. So, for example, we might question why it is that many groups are forming at the present time to learn about and collectively find the support to manage individual life experiences of caring for family members with dementia. The answer to this might lie in increasing longevity due to advances in medical science and technology, the withdrawal of government provision in social and health care, and so on. The important point to note here is that group workers must recognise the significance of the temporal period in which the group is contextualised. This may mean that group workers directly address these issues within the group—for example, drawing attention to the effect of social structures in marginalising or stigmatising individuals—or that they are alert to the political dimensions of the personal issues which the group may have been established to meet—for example, recognising that the perceived and actual burden of caring for a disabled family member has policy implications beyond the immediate experience.

The purpose of this chapter is to provide approaches to understanding the life of the group and in so doing to give us a road map or a guide to the likely or possible routes which groups may take. Our primary interest here is to think about what happens to, and within, a group over time and how we, as leaders, organisers, facilitators or participants, might use this understanding to shape, sustain and think about the group. It is the passage of time and the character of the historical period which provide both the context and the impetus for the group's work.

Within the Western philosophical and cultural tradition, one of the oldest themes concerns the subject of time. Two 'eternal metaphors' (Gould 1988, p. 199) prevail: the concept of time's arrow and time's cycle. The metaphor of time's arrow refers to the understanding of history as an irreversible sequence of unrepeatable events in which each moment occupies its own distinctive position in a temporal series. All of these moments are linked in a sequence which has a direction, and is moving towards some end. Time's arrow thus presupposes that phenomena will be transformed through the passage of time and, with adequate study, this progression can be understood. On the other hand, the metaphor of time's cycle provides an image of events as without meaning and without direction. Fundamental states are immanent in time, continuously present and unchanging. The impression of change might be conveyed through the appearance of movement, but in fact such movements are rather cycles which are repeated precisely and exactly. Time's cycle thus refers to a state of timeless order characterised by immanent law-like structures (see Gould 1988, Ch. 1).

For most of us, notions of time commensurate with the time's arrow metaphor are taken for granted. As Flaherty (1999, p. 1) points out: 'The fundamental quality of duration is embedded in our impression that things are not as they were before; that is that things have changed.' In fact, we rarely question the veracity of our observations of the biological world in which time seems synonymous with change: infants are born, grow and develop into adults, then decline as they age until death occurs. When we look at the way theorists, practitioners and participants talk about the group experience, similar perspectives are obvious: the group is seen as if it were a living thing with a life characterised by growth, development and change. Directly or indirectly, the concept of time is a central organising principle of group work. Importantly, however, human beings are not passive or merely 'acted on' by the passage of time. Rather, they make use of time as a resource by, for example, being selective in what they pay attention to. Time, then, is both the impetus for and the context within which the group's purpose is achieved.

Seeing time in this way—as a primary organising element of the group—suggests that it is important to draw a distinction between the two basic types of groups discussed in Chapter 7: open ongoing groups, and closed time-limited groups. With ongoing open groups, particularly restitution and recapitulation groups and sometimes support and rehabilitation groups, the time available for the group is potentially infinite. The group has a beginning with some members but others join it at different points. So individuals (generally in consultation and negotiation with their fellow participants and the leader) enact their own time-frames. In an important sense, they create their own group as dictated by their needs as they perceive them. At one moment in the group's life, a member might be terminating involvement whilst another is commencing. This stands in marked contrast to the closed time-limited group, in particular task and action groups and growth and education groups, which by definition exist within a predetermined time-frame which is usually shared by all members—they begin and conclude their involvement collectively.

Let us look more closely at the way in which the concept of time is understood by group work theorists, practitioners and participants.

TheOrists

In conceptualising the relation between time and change, theorists have tended to concentrate their attention on time-limited groups and to propose that such groups can be understood as developing in certain predictable ways—essentially as the time's arrow metaphor would suggest. Given that the group is structured at the outset to conclude at a predetermined point, it is logical to propose that such structuring will have implications for what happens. Clearly there is a limit imposed on the amount of time available in which the group's purpose is to be achieved. Knowing this in advance imposes pressure. (As has been said in another context, the thought of an ending 'wonderfully concentrates the mind'!) Such pressure may mean that participants will be expected (or will expect themselves) to focus their efforts to overcome perceived or actual barriers to the achievement of their aims. An outcome of this may be seen in the emergence of anxiety and conflict as well as concerted efforts to work collaboratively. To this factor (the time-limited structure of the group) we can, to some extent, attribute the apparent consensus found in many accounts of group stages and phases of development. Despite other differences, such as the type of group and the issues or needs it is designed to address, common phases of development are described.

The ways in which time-limited groups are expected to develop have been understood either as: (a) recurring in a linear stage-by-stage sequence, each stage building on the previous or (b) non-linear phases that represent group processes as moving from phase to phase and returning to various phases as time elapses. For example, many of us are familiar with Tuckman's (1963) description of the linear sequence in groups of forming, storming, norming, performing and adjourning. In his account, group participants can be observed to move from polite and tentative exchanges at the beginning to conflict and a testing-out to establish themselves in the group. This is a precursor to the formation of trust and bonding which will enable the work of the group to take place prior to its termination.

Corey (2000, pp. 87–135) has proposed six stages which, while very similar to Tuckman's, include two 'bookends'. The first is *formation*, which begins before the group meets and includes the process of selecting and recruiting members. The second comprises *follow-up and evaluation*, where Corey advocates providing a post-group follow-up and evaluation meeting to ensure that gains achieved in the group are identified and maintained.

Brower (1996), while still adhering to a linear time's arrow conceptualisation of group development, offers an alternative perspective, noting how members construct their experiences differently over time. He posits, drawing on personal construct theory, that groups move from a state of anomie or structurelessness which creates a crisis for members in trying to make sense of their experience. Out of their anxiety, they initially turn to the group leader for help and may, for a time, adopt the leader's version of what the group means. However, over time they begin to question the leader's version and turn to themselves to develop their own shared version of the meaning of the group. It is on the basis of this 'shared schema' that members confront problems and negotiate their group passage together.

Most theorists argue that each of these stages or phases offers developmental challenges which groups must deal with, but not necessarily resolve, if they are to move on to the next stage. However, elements of other stages may reappear in subsequent stages as the group weaves its way towards achieving its purpose in what could be described as a pendular, rather than linear, movement (Berman-Rossi 1992).

Manor (2000), whose perspective on systems theory was described in Chapter 3, proposes that groups evolve through eight stages (2000, p. 86). These stages are marked by phases and crises which will differ in respect of the way particular groups construct their progress. Crises occur when group members experience ambivalence about the group's move to a subsequent phase. For example, in stage 5, the 'Intimacy Crisis' (2000, pp. 144–70), group members are challenged to deal with personal issues stirred by the content of the group's discussion. The ensuing crisis revolves around their own ambivalent wishes to reveal vulnerabilities and still be accepted by others. Resolution of this crisis—a redrawing of personal and interpersonal boundaries created by entering a different level of involvement—enables the group to progress to the next phase. Central to Manor's perspective is the concept of the group as a communication cycle 'driven' by a dynamic combination of process, structure and contents (2000, p. 63). Manor is critical of various theorists' attempts to identify stages because of their failure to account for differences in groups and the tendency for such frameworks to be overly prescriptive. His own contribution is an attempt to account for differences and commonalities by proposing a framework which, in his view, is flexible, inclusive and comprehensive (2000, p. 66).

Most descriptions of group phases and stages assume gender neutrality—that all groups will evolve and develop through phases and stages irrespective of the gender of participants. However, Hagen (1983) and Schiller (1997) (see also Cohn 1996; Bernardez 1996) offer a similar but alternative viewpoint. Schiller argues, on the basis of feminist understandings of the primary importance to women of connection and affiliation, that women's groups can be conceptualised as moving through five stages.

While the first (pre-affiliation) and final (termination) stages are common to all groups, the middle phases in women's groups differ in that conflict occurs later. Schiller (1997) argues that the importance of establishing a safe relational base precedes the exploration and recognition of difference (stage 3)—'members are able to allow and appreciate each other's differences within the framework of their affiliation and connection' (1997, p. 5). This is a necessary precursor to the negotiation of conflict for, without strong empathic bonds and the assurance of safety, the management of conflict in productive and constructive ways will be inhibited. Schiller's point (1997, p. 10) is that, for many women, engagement in conflict while still maintaining the connection is a particularly challenging issue. She comments on the logic of conflict thus occurring later in women's groups:

Rather than jumping into the area of greatest difficulty first, that of dealing with conflict, authority and power, women first set the stage with what they do well: giving support, bonding around common issues, and generally not challenging each other or the facilitator directly early on.

Janet draws a comparison between single session focus groups with men-only and women-only participants: *'One focus group of five men . . . it turned into a territorial battle . . . we hadn't had that with the women's group.'* If Schiller's theorisation is correct and Janet had organised a number of focus groups, conflict may have emerged at a later point in the women's group.

In conversation with Bridget about her group, the Women's Circus, she too emphasised the importance of women feeling safe in the group, especially where group participants may have experienced sexual abuse. The achievement of a sense of safety has occurred over time, and with it a perception that the group has developed and matured. Bridget says:

The whole body of the Circus has matured . . . we used to wear white faces on the stage and that made it safe to go out there because it was quite hard to tell who you were and there would be lots of scenes with lots of women on stage. So we've learned by doing that. The Artistic Director said 'now it is a mature body and we don't need the white mask' and now we're using our voices more and we never used to before . . . it's as though the body has matured and found its voice . . .

So far in this discussion we have been focusing on groups whose purposes are therapeutic, supportive or educational, such as recapitulation and restitution groups, growth and education groups, and support and rehabilitation groups. Task and action groups (which include community development groups), while differing from those with a clinical or interpersonal focus, have been understood as developing stages or phases reminiscent of the mutual aid model (see Shulman 1999;

Garland et al. 1973). Mondros and Berman-Rossi (1991) argue that task and action groups tend to focus attention on content and action strategies rather than on interpersonal or 'here and now' issues in the group.

This tendency arises out of a key characteristic of such groups— that is, that organisers of social action or community development groups see their overriding purpose as being to empower people and to redistribute existing power. This perspective means that the organiser will see their role as firstly to help participants act on their own behalf, and secondly to redistribute power. As people gain strength and a sense of competence, they will then organise to pursue their own interests. The organiser assists in working with them to establish a viable organisation which will be the power base from which participants are able to negotiate with other power holders. However, Mondros and Berman-Rossi (1991) propose that organisers of such groups must be alert to what happens in the group. A tendency with task and action groups is to assume that it is the issue itself around which members have organised that is primary. Without an understanding of the likely stages of group development, organisers may misinterpret conflict, difference in opinion and challenges as detrimental to the group's purpose. Where the emergence of these elements is understood as a neces- sary and usual aspect of the life of any group, organisers will anticipate and make use of them rather than attempt to avoid conflict and dissension by overly controlling the group. In conver- sation with Helen, she made a similar point with regard to her social action group:

If you bring people together you have to hold it together and therefore there has to be some shared understanding of what's happening and where each person's coming from . . . you need enough overlap [between the goal and what is happening in the group] to suit the particular group.

147

The many writers who address the issue of stages and phases in the life of the group are all emphatic in pointing out that these are not present in every group, nor do they occur in the particular order identified. Groups may weave and cycle amongst them in different ways and to different degrees. In addition, it is important to recognise that once we acknowledge the centrality of time as an organising principle in group work, the time-limited group is recognised as having a beginning and an end. Ebenstein (1998, p. 51) argues that even in single-session groups which are one-off meetings for one to two hours, similar stages can be observed. The group has its own beginning, middle and end requiring the leader's attention. The life of the group is what can be thought of as 'filling the spaces' between and incorporating the beginning and the end. Indeed, beginnings and endings are not even as clear-cut as this suggests: in the minds and memories of participants, where their involvement began and ended lies in their interpretation of what a group has meant to them. For some, the ending of a group may become a point of departure rather than closure.

Practitioners

Action in the group exists within time and the originator of the group—generally the designated leader—proposes the time-frame at the outset. The belief is that this time will be 'enough' for the various group processes they anticipate will occur in order to achieve the group's purpose and the desired change. In other words, the leader acknowledges that it takes time to process the information brought into the group as well as that generated in participants' subjective responses to the group situation itself. The leader has a role in enabling participants to bring the internal and the shared experiences together through facilitating members' involvement and interaction as the group processes ebb and flow. We can identify three approaches which group workers may take:

1   practitioners who closely structure time and 'interrupt' it with the introduction of particular kinds of input which will prompt the change required. This is the belief underpinning growth and education groups and some support and rehabilitation groups. These 'interruptions' may take the form of didactic input, videos, role-plays, artwork, and so on;

2   practitioners who specify the end or the target of the group—for example the production of a report or the holding of elections by a certain date and time—and devise strategies in relation to that. Task and action groups, and some self-help groups, are structured in this way;

3   practitioners who use time itself as the context within which the processes that are the focus of the group's work will occur. Recapitulation and restitution groups reflect this kind of conceptualisation of time, as do some support and rehabilitation groups which are open-ended and unstructured. For example, in a group which is time-unlimited, the annual four-week break at Christmas may be experienced as stressful and anxiety-provoking for some participants. The meaning of this period when the group does not meet, when there is 'no time' for the group, will need exploration and interpretation to assist participants in managing the impact of absence and separation highlighted by a change in the usual time-frame.

Group participants

Group participants also have their own views about time and its relation to change. Their personal time-frames may be set by the conditions of their lives (work and family commitments, mobility, health), the pressing nature of the problem or issue and the priority it assumes in their emotional or political needs hierarchy. In addition, their beliefs about the relationship between time and change will make a difference to their experience, for instance: how long they believe is 'long enough' for the group experience to impact usefully on them and their beliefs about the kind of group experience that they desire—for example, a psychoeducational (structured and short-term) as opposed to a psychoanalytic (open, long-term) group experience. What we are referring to here is group participants' subjective experience of time—that is, the ways in which they construct the meaning that time holds within their conceptualisation of the group and its relationship to their daily lives.

Group processes

However we view the time–change coupling, group workers are focused on the processes as they occur during—or indeed may come to comprise—the experience of leading and participating in a group. The work of the group takes place within the time made available (it being a particular form of temporal experience), and this in turn determines the way in which the group work is done, what happens and what does not happen.

The work of the group is reflected in the processes which occur. These processes are enacted primarily through talk, through telling stories, doing activities collectively, reflecting on these events and moments, trying to make sense of them, and using them strategically in order to achieve both the group's purpose and the purposes individual members bring with them.

The talk, the games or tasks, the engagement or disengagement and the thinking and reflecting together that make up the experience of group processes may be conceptualised and interpreted from different theoretical standpoints (see Chapter 3). Shulman (1999) refers to processes as those elements which create and sustain the group as a mutual aid system—for example, through sharing data, discussing taboo areas, individual problem-solving, and so on. Manor (2000, p. 94), also from a systems perspective, describes processes as 'types of feedback that connect people with one another . . . amplifying, symbolising, and clarifying'. Dean (1998) identifies group processes as emerging through the stories that are told and the narratives constructed to give meaning to experience. Yalom (1975) refers to 'curative factors', such as the instillation of hope, interpersonal learning, altruism and catharsis, as ways of naming group processes. They refer to interpersonal transactions between (in Yalom's language) therapist and patient which comprise verbal utterances, the meaning of which is derived from the 'how' and the 'why' of the patient's words (1975, pp. 122–23):

the 'how' and the 'why' illuminate some aspects of the patient's relationship to others with whom he [sic] is interacting. Thus, the therapist considers the metacommunicational aspects of the message. Why, from the relationship aspect, is the patient making the statement at this time, to this person, in this manner?

In task and action groups, group processes are contained in the decisions, strategies and tactics members devise to achieve their collective goals.

Thus very similar events and activities (talk, actions, tasks, exchange and communication with others) are interpreted differently in relation to one's theoretical perspective, the way issues are problematised and theorised, and their representation in the espoused purpose identified for each group.

This underlines the fact that, although groups may be formed for a great range of purposes and although they may take a variety of forms, their common characteristic is that they create processes— in other words, some things happen and other things do not happen when a collection of people get together. Group workers must heighten their awareness of these processes. Group processes can be understood as occurring around and emphasising two central preoccupations of group participants: with power and with resources.

Power and resources

In Chapter 5 we explored the concept of power in groups as the capacity to influence what happens in the group—that is, to influence processes which enact the work of the group: what will be done, how it will be done, what can happen and what cannot happen. Power inheres in the relationships of members and leaders in groups, and it is these relationships which enable action (of any kind) to take place or to be inhibited.

Central to this capacity to influence (to empower or disempower), are the resources which members and leaders bring to the group. These resources refer to skills, knowledge, experience, time and availability, as well as emotional resources of care, concern, energy, empathy, commitment and moral support. The extent to which these resources become available to the group is evidenced by the degree of cohesion, bonding, solidarity—and their counterpart, trust—which emerge as the group works together. A key indicator of the extent to which cohesion has developed in the group is in the emergence of conflict and the capacity for the group to survive and prosper from its occurrence. No group can exist without conflict, but not all groups survive its appearance and not all groups recognise its presence. The presence of conflict signals that the group has begun to matter to its members—that they have engaged with one another and the leader. Power relationships emerge as re-negotiable and sometimes this re-negotiation happens through conflict. Conflict also signals that they are struggling with a central dilemma of all groups: how to meet individual needs for recognition of difference and autonomy in the context of collective strivings to which they are also committed. Bridget notes:

> If you have a problem with someone else in the circus you try and deal with it with them . . . [we need to] deal with conflict, accept that conflict is likely to occur at some time . . . it's accepted that there will be upsets and we'll work them out . . .

Over the life of the group, participants are constantly changing as they perceive, understand and respond to what happens in the group. They may move from a position of anxiety and perceived powerlessness to one in which they recognise both the barriers to, and the opportunities for, greater autonomy and influence within the group. These changed perceptions are related to the passage of time in the group as members negotiate together and struggle with their anxieties and doubts, finding common ground, differences, discomfort and challenge along the path to achieving both the group's and their own individual purposes.

We noted in Chapter 5 that one of the resources the leader brings to the group is knowledge and experience. If we consider that the leader knows something of the ways in which groups evolve over time, this presupposes that they will be in a position to recognise and antic-ipate likely stages or phases which chart the group's course. At different moments, the leader will interpret what happens as relevant to the kind of group (time-limited or time-unlimited), the character-istics of participants, the group's purpose and the length of time it has been meeting. The stage or phase which characterises the group's development thus calls for different leader interventions. It also indicates which aspects of the power–resources struggle preoccupy the group.

It is useful to describe this process in broad terms of beginning, middle and end phases. Such a 'broad brush' approach to group stages clearly cannot account for the particular variations of individual groups. Rather, this depiction is intended to be somewhat vague and indistinct, approximating the 'lived experience' of participating in a group. Indeed, such stages and phases are more likely to be identified in retrospect. As such, they can be helpful conceptual tools for finding order in the complexity of the group process. However, to use them prescriptively may interrupt and overly control the group's 'natural' life. Importantly too, considering time-limited groups have begin-nings, middles and ends retains the conceptual and actual relationship between time and the group's life. By keeping this relationship in mind, group workers (and participants) may be better able to pace themselves in relation to what they want to achieve in their time together. Maintaining this connection between time and change reinforces workers' and participants' own agency with regard to making use of time, rather than seeing the group as a kind of juggernaut rolling forward on its own trajectory.

Beginning phase

Members join the group with varying levels of anxiety, fear, hope and anticipation. They do not know one another, but they do know the espoused group purpose. These factors suggest that the leader may respond to those issues by enabling members to begin to get to know one another. Some leaders organise 'getting to know you' exercises as icebreakers (see Benjamin et al. 1997); others prefer not to dissolve anxiety too soon, seeing it as an important force in galvanising participants' engagement (see Kaplan and Saddock 1971, Ch. 1). This beginning phase is characterised by the participants' endeavours to find common ground together which will build a sense of safety, cohesion and trust. An aspect of discovering common ground lies in a revisiting of the espoused group purpose, exploring its relevance to the individual agendas of participants. Conflict and tension may also be apparent here as participants strive to find their place in the group, to discover how they can exert influence on what happens, and how they can manage the tension that arises when differences and divergent styles and personalities become known. The leader's role here is to offer interpretations to participants about what he/she understands is happening; enabling members to draw meaning from the events which, in turn, strengthens and empowers them.

> We use the environment that develops in the group . . . it's not a therapy group. I introduce it as a time for women for themselves

because that's one of the things women are most poor in—time for themselves. (Heather)

I provide the role-modelling in terms of respectful listening, not being racist, sexist, put-down or patronising . . . (Chris)

Good performance hangs on a good process. Process right from the beginning has an edge about 'you're here to do things—you're not in a counselling group. (Bridget)

Middle phase

The group leader may be less active at this point, as the arrival of the middle phase is marked by a sense of stability and of participants having negotiated a way in which they can and wish to work together to achieve the group's purpose. The leader may provide the group with alternative explanations for their observations or alternative strategies for how they might act. He/she may draw on similar resources of knowledge and experience which members themselves bring. Such tactics are effective in devolving power to members by recognising their expertise and reinforcing their capacity to contribute to the group's progress.

. . . getting them [the men] to think and ask questions about their own stuff and see their own stuff differently . . . (Chris)

Sometimes participants [are] better at picking up when a participant has had negative experiences than we [the group leaders] are. (Heather)

As the group evolves and they start to get used to the group environment . . . they find that they do learn from each other in different ways . . . learning about the commonality of experience and measuring themselves . . . they can somehow measure where they're at and how they're going [in a way] that they can't get from the leaders. (Robyn)

We just meet and tend to discuss what we want but there is somebody there if we do get a bit off the track . . . they're observing us rather than actually leading. They do get us back on track if need be. (Breast Cancer Therapy Group)

Even though I mightn't be speaking or talking about myself, just sitting quietly and listening to somebody else speaking and think— 'oh, that person is saying he or she reacts like that—how do I react?' . . . some of the most valuable things I've got out of the group have been through listening to others. (Bernard)

The leader puts questions back to the group—'What do you think?' That encourages us to explore, which is very good. (Breast Cancer Therapy Group)

I know that all of it is manageable [yet] sometimes it gets very overwhelming but you just take it a step at a time. It's all manageable, you access resources . . . (Maria)

End phase

In time-limited groups, because the time available for the group's work is running out, the leader's role is to work to enable participants to maximise their gains from earlier work in the group. This may be done by encouraging a reflective mode amongst participants, placing greater emphasis on participants' capacity to observe and think about what is happening. In time-limited groups, as the final meetings of the group approach, the leader needs to be alert to the extent to which members are able to detach themselves from the group and take what gains they have made with them. This may mean that the leader is more active than in the middle phase, encouraging the members to evaluate their experience and identify strategies for moving on outside the group. Members may begin to feel apprehensive about the end of the group and time must be made available for feelings of loss or disappointment to be worked with. In the following quotes from group workers and participants, we see the ways in which speakers are able to reflect on the progress that they (or the group) have made or are making, and the kinds of gains that the group experience has given them.

> They feel they've got skills and a knowledge base that can equip them . . . (Robyn)

> I no longer take the crap because I had people listening to me . . . I'll never be the same because of it—I'm much more assertive and smarter. (Maria)

> The leader puts a constant emphasis on you doing it. He says— 'therapy doesn't get you better, you get yourself better.' It's what you learn—therapy is about wisdom, knowledge of yourself and I suppose he's right. He says— 'if you get yourself better in therapy it's not my doing, it's you—you did it yourself'. (Bernard)

Taking another perspective on the leader's role over the life of the group, Burkhardt (1982, p. 163) draws attention to the impact of the social and political context on the group's development. He argues that, in social action groups, the shifts occurring in wider society will alter the dynamics of the group's processes. The organiser (a term more appropriate to this form of group work than 'leader'), always moving between focusing on the personal and political dimensions of the group's life, will 'read' the external climate and act accordingly. So, for instance, in a conservative political climate where the success of collective action may be doubtful, attention may need to be placed on political perspectives to 'counter the overattention to personal and technical matters' which may begin to dominate the group. In a more 'progressive' era when the social action group is driven by a strong political and social focus and is imbued with a belief that collective action will be successful, the organiser may have to ensure that the personal dimensions of the issue at stake and its impact on their daily lives receive attention.

The phases or stages we have discussed which mark the progress of the group are, as was noted earlier, more perceptible in time-limited groups. However, in computer-mediated collaborative work, quite different issues with regard to time arise, given that communication is not face-to-face and is often not synchronous (for further discussion, see McGrath and Berdahl 1998).

Where the group is open-ended—for example, in an ongoing issue-focused group such as Bob's or a long-term psychotherapy group such as Bernard's—time is differently understood. In these types of groups, individuals themselves organise how they use the time available. The group may be seen as going through the same kinds of phases or stages identified in relation to time-limited groups, but as the group is not intended to conclude, these phases or stages will be understood differently. So, for instance, conflict and challenge over positions of power and influence in the group, or anxieties and tensions related to fears about the availability of resources, will be recognised as referring to ongoing struggles that are the hallmark of all human enterprises. In this sense, they are not necessarily seen as being 'forced' by the time-limited nature of the group. This distinction has implications for how the group works when these struggles emerge. Where they are seen as synonymous with collective work, the focus of members may be directed to unconscious elements of individual and collective life, including those aspects which may be outside immediate awareness and emanate from 'wider' political, social and economic factors. In contrast, where the group is time-limited, attention may be focused on how the finite and predetermined structure of the group affects the emotional responses of group members—for example, in adding pressure on them to understand or resolve something quickly, or the impending loss of newly established bonds with others.

Summary

To sum up, we can draw out several important issues for working with groups from a consideration of the temporal nature of group work:

- Time-limited and time-unlimited groups are conceptualised differently with reference to time and hence have different practice implications.
- In time-limited groups, particular phases and stages have been noted as characterising the group's progress from inception to conclusion. The identification of stages and phases is a reflection of the structured nature of the group and the impact this has on both the participants' emotional responses and on the practical outcomes—for example, learning and understanding—that can occur.
- All collective human enterprises are centrally preoccupied with the distribution of power and the availability of resources. Groups are no exception. In the time-limited group, these preoccupations and their emergence in conflict or disagreement are understood as, in part, being due to the effects of temporal structure—that is, because the group is to end these events and press for resolution.
- In the time-unlimited group, the distribution of power and resources is identified as continuous and ongoing, and best understood with reference to the influence of unconscious elements and those 'wider' political and social factors outside the group impacting upon and influencing relationships inside the group. The focus of the group will be to explore and understand them, rather than to resolve them. They are not so much impediments but rather important 'windows' into understanding the way social and emotional life influences, and is influenced by, collective and individual action.

When a group worker decides to establish a group, the implications of the temporal structure need consideration. If the group is time-limited, the understandings available to us about what is likely to happen from the beginning to the end can, to an extent, be planned for. This is where knowledge of the likely phases and stages the group will progress through can enable us to prepare for particular events, such as conflict or feelings of loss, to emerge at different points. In the time-unlimited group, how sense is made of similar emotional responses will more often refer to theoretical understanding related to our knowledge of unconscious mental life and the impact of structural factors on the group.

However, the key question for group workers and participants working with both time-limited and time-unlimited groups is how the group can best make use of the time available to achieve its espoused and emergent purposes. The different ways in which this question can be answered in different types of groups are apparent in the following comments.

Robyn, referring to a structured six week psychoeducational group says:

[The leader] needs to carry an understanding of what the group's purpose is for today: why are we meeting? Is there a good match between my agenda and their agenda? There [needs to be] a delicate balance between content and process.

Maria, in reference to her ongoing self-help and advocacy group, says: 'You're in it for the long haul and for life . . .', while Bernard, a participant in an open psychoanalytically oriented psychotherapy group, reflects:

It doesn't really have a structure . . . there isn't a sense of time being divided among members of the group . . . the group takes on a life of its own and I just go along with it but if I want to I could leave—you're always free to come back.

CRITICAL ISSUES:
'It's a bit of a risk . . . you just don't know what will happen'

This chapter is about the kinds of critical issues which characterise work with groups. As we saw earlier in this book, the group leader, working collaboratively with participants, has several tasks—chief amongst them that of working to keep the group cohesive and united so that its purpose and the purposes of members can be achieved. Group leaders bring resources to the group, resources comprised of knowledge, skills, energy and the capacity to 'think group'. Group members also bring elements of these resources (and others). The group worker's role includes making the openings possible so that participants can contribute to and benefit from this pooling of resources. When difficulties and challenges arise, these present opportunities for the worker to resource the group. Simultaneously, they make up the life of the group, reflecting the dilemmas and tensions which characterise the coming together of individual pressure to meet needs, and the collective need of the group. So, rather than considering these challenges as 'interruptions' to an otherwise smooth-flowing process, they exemplify and embody that process.

In this chapter, several issues will be described, with examples depicting likely scenarios which may pose challenges. These particular issues have been chosen (out of all the possible issues) because they were frequently raised in my conversations with leaders and participants. Many of them have also been studied in research and texts on group work. A brief discussion of them will be presented, highlighting the themes or issues which are of relevance in deciding what to do to maximise the potential of incidents or moments for the group's advancement. We shall look at:

- the first meeting of the group;
- a new member joining the group;
- a member's decision to leave;
- conflict:
  - member to member;
  - member to worker;
- the silent member;
- the dominating member;
- the uncooperative group;
- the final meeting.

The examples used to illustrate these issues are fictitious and do not refer to actual groups.

The first meeting of the group

The first time I was terrified . . . that was really quite daunting . . . (Breast Cancer Therapy Group)

The first time coming into a group and the thought of walking into a group of strangers—it's pretty daunting . . . (Bernard)

For some it's not an easy process, coming to and staying in the group. (Lou)

For all group workers and most group members, the first meeting of the group is a very important event (see McCallum 1997). All participants may come to the first meeting with a mixture of anxiety and expectation. Some of the questions they may be asking themselves might be:

- What am I supposed to do?
- What do I want? Why did I decide to come along?
- Will the group give me what I want?
- What will it be like?
- Will others like me?
- Will I like the others?
- Will I like the leader?
- Will the leader like me?

In addition the group worker may be asking him/herself:

- How will I manage things and establish the group firmly enough so that they'll come back next week?
- How should I present myself?
- Will I need to get them talking to one another?
- How do I stop them talking at the end of the session?
- What will I do if someone takes over and dominates?
- What will I do if there is a fight or someone gets upset?
- What if they ignore or attack me?
- How much control should I exert?

Being aware of these mixed emotions evoked by the first meeting is important (see McCallum 1997). Depending on the type of group, its purpose, the characteristics of members and the worker's style of doing things, there are a number of ways to begin this process of working together. For most groups, the worker's main purpose is to put in place the opportunities for members to begin to talk with one another and establish areas of shared interest or common ground. This is important in building trust and working towards establishing some

163

cohesion. Some leaders like to structure the first meeting with group games or getting-to-know-you activities (see Benjamin et al. 1997, Ch. 6; Ivey et al. 2001). Others use the first meeting (particularly in a psychoeducational group) to explore the proposed program and use this somewhat intellectual discussion as an opportunity for members to introduce their interests and concerns in a relatively neutral fashion (see Shulman 1999, Ch. 10). Others, particularly those working with long-term psychotherapy groups, prefer to allow members to find their own ways of communicating with others, believing that people are ready to join emotionally at different times, the first meeting being only part of this process (see Yalom 1975, Ch. 10).

Example 1

A mutual aid group for women with a terminal illness was designed as an open group. While members would join and leave throughout the duration of the group, the first meeting began with seven women. Each woman had been interviewed briefly prior to the group meeting by the co-leaders. The purpose of this interview was to meet her and for her to meet the leaders, to check whether she was still willing to join and whether she understood what would be involved, to let her know the group guidelines such as confidentiality and to answer any questions she may have about the group. This preliminary meeting also began the process of engaging her with the group. The group meetings were scheduled for an hour-and-a-half and were held in a meeting room which belonged to the social work department of a large metropolitan hospital. On the day of the first scheduled meeting, most of the women assembled in the waiting room about ten minutes ahead of time. When the co-leaders invited them into the meeting room, they were already talking animatedly together and had exchanged names. Once seated in the group circle, there was a brief, anxious silence. This was short lived when one member, Julie, suggested that they could all briefly tell a bit about their experience of the illness. The discussion took off energetically. The women talked about the major disruption to their lives that the diagnosis had meant, the importance of finding friends who cared and were not afraid of the disease, and the recognition that their identity as women, workers, mothers and friends was of far greater significance than the identity of 'patient' allowed them. At the end of the meeting, there was discussion about coming back the next week, and the suggestion that Kaye would bring some information she had accessed on the internet to share with them. When the meeting finished, several women decided to go and have coffee together. The co-leaders had taken a rather low profile during this meeting. Their interventions were reflections on what was happening as they observed the women reaching out to one another, encouraging a quiet member 'in', finding things in common. The co-leaders saw their role primarily as facilitating the women's own capacities to establish contact with one another, for the women to control the group towards meeting their own needs while providing a boundary and a containment for the members' explorations.

Example 2

A social action group concerned to prevent the opening of their quiet cul-de-sac to traffic visiting a facility for disabled people located at the end of the street met in the home of Dr W. Prior to this meeting, all neighbours had received notification of the facility's intention to apply for a planning permit to change the street. There had been considerable discussion amongst neighbours when the notice arrived and the decision to meet was spontaneous. Dr W offered his home for the first meeting. Beforehand, he and his neighbour, Jim, an accountant, had put together an agenda. When everyone arrived they were served drinks by Mrs W and collected in the lounge room. Dr W welcomed people and circulated copies of the agenda. Discussion was noisy and heated and Dr W found himself asserting a leadership role, calling for order and structuring the meeting so everyone could have a say. After about two hours, Jim suggested they devise an action plan. A decision-making structure requiring a majority vote was agreed to and Dr W and Jim were put forward by the group as leaders and spokespersons. By the end of the meeting, a plan containing various strategies was in place and the next meeting had been organised, at which time these strategies would be put to the vote. It was decided that the meeting would again be at Dr W's house. Neighbours went home feeling positive with what they had achieved and seemed pleased to have Dr W and Jim as leaders.

Example 3

A psychoeducational group was formed for adolescents aged between fourteen and eighteen years who had a parent living with schizophrenia. The purpose of the group was to provide information about the nature of schizophrenia, the likely impact on family life and strategies for dealing with problems that might arise for young people in this situation. Very importantly, the group worker wanted this group to provide opportunities for young people to make contact with peers, sharing their own experiences and building supportive bonds with one another. The group was designed to have eight meetings of two hours' duration and to combine educational information with activities and discussion. Participants in this age group were invited to join by the case managers in a community mental health clinic who were familiar with the family make-up of their principal clients, the parents with schizophrenia. The group worker, Terry, spoke to each of them on the phone but decided against a formal pre-meeting assessment as he felt this might make his role more that of an authority figure than he thought would be helpful.

Terry carefully planned and structured the group program, scheduling meetings in the late afternoon and booking a meeting room in a centrally located neighbourhood house rather than the clinic. The neighbourhood house was adjacent to basketball courts and a sports field.

Eight young people, four males and four females, attended the first meeting. None had met before. Terry provided coloured pens, paper and various humorous stickers for them to use to make their own individualised name tags. Soft drinks and biscuits were available for them to have as they arrived. The room had an assortment of arm chairs and bean bags and Terry asked them to 'grab a seat' and draw it into the circle. He briefly sketched out the purpose of the group and how he proposed to schedule input and activities for the next seven meetings; warmly encouraging participants to put forward other ideas or suggestions which occurred to them as time went by. He outlined what he called 'ground rules' for the group—for example, that people would come on time and would let him know if they had to miss a meeting so no one would worry if they were absent. Terry then turned to introductions, beginning with himself and his personal experience as a young person, noting that this did not include having a parent with schizophrenia, and his interest in young people and mental health issues.

The participants had said very little so far, so Terry invited each of them to give their name and to answer the question: What do I want to get out of this group? With their permission, he wrote their answers on separate pieces of butcher's paper, telling them that they would review these initial comments at the last meeting to check how well their early wishes had been met.

The next half hour was spent outside on the basketball court messing around with a 'shooting for goal' activity. The group reconvened for a debriefing, with each participant offering one sentence about 'what they had learned' at that meeting. Terry briefly sketched what he had in mind for the next session the following week.

Discussion

These rather different examples highlight various factors of importance in the first group meeting:

- *The group worker(s)'s need to be clear on the group's purpose:* in the first case, the purpose was primarily for the women to establish networks of care and support with one another and to find a contained space to express feelings; in the social action case, the group's purpose was to come up with an action strategy. In the adolescent group, it was to combine information with building support amongst participants to relieve isolation and increase the range of possible strategies they could learn from one another in handling potentially difficult family issues.

- *The need to prepare:* the co-leaders of the women's group had worked together for many years and were familiar with one another's styles of working and were clear about the purpose of the group and its theoretical framework. Even so, they had talked beforehand about how they planned to lead the group and were prepared, should it not happen spontaneously, to invite each member to share a little of her experience as a beginning point. (As it turned out, this was not necessary.) In the social action group, members had not worked together before but they did know each other. Preparation in this group involved devising an agenda in order to keep the group focused. In the adolescent group, the group worker, Terry, had prepared extensively. He was aware of the age of participants and the likely psychosocial developmental stage they were working through. He was also aware that issues to do with establishing a sense of identity and direction in life and a desire for independence were of significance to the participants but that this might be coupled with insecurity and awkwardness. Terry used this knowledge in planning the group by, for example, structuring the meeting so there would be a firm focus, using specific and clear questions to get participants talking, offering a mixture of activities from sitting, listening and talking to socialising and playing together.

- For many psychotherapeutic and psychoeducational groups, it is useful to meet beforehand with prospective members in order to get to know the member's individual stories a little, to introduce the leader(s) to the prospective members, and to be alerted to any particular issues which an individual may bring. This allows the group worker(s) to anticipate potential sensitivities or problems indicated by the individual's history and thus handle them in the group should they arise (see Shulman 1999, pp. 337–40; Ch. 11). The social action group in this example comprised people who already knew something about each other and may have been able to anticipate areas of difference. However, the clear task focus put these aspects on the 'back burner'. By way of contrast, in the young people's group, participants had not met in person with the group worker beforehand because Terry was emphatic that this might increase the sense of his (the group worker's) greater authority. He believed that this could be detrimental in a group of adolescents and wanted to establish a more collegial atmosphere from the start. Terry's use of self-disclosure in the first meeting and his attention to ensuring that the setting for the group was as informal as possible were strategies to complement his belief.

- In a psychoeducational or psychotherapeutic group, it is especially important to recognise the mixture of anticipatory and anxious emotions that come with the first meeting and, where appropriate, to comment on these in the group. This is an important aspect of establishing an empathic and understanding climate within the group as well as containing any anxiety in a constructive way. The social action group also met for the first time about an issue of considerable emotional and practical concern to them. The decision to begin by serving drinks and trying to establish a convivial climate was a strategic way to engage people around the common issues. As the group met in Dr W's home, there may have been a sense that he was offering himself as a leader. His hospitality may have been intended to encourage such a view at the same time as it reinforced the sense of 'neighbourliness' which was so important to the success of the proposed campaign. In the young people's group, the group worker was focused on lessening anxieties and encouraging talking. The order in which he planned the meeting was designed to do this—for example, by requiring little of the participants at the outset. Terry also used modelling in introducing himself first and disclosing some personal details as a way of indicating what could be both relevant and safe to say in the group.

A new member joining the group

Sometimes we need to remind ourselves that someone who's just joined does not have the knowledge or the history but brings an equal contribution in skills and energy. (Bridget)

It's sometimes a bit hard for the group to accept newcomers . . . (Heather)

Example

A mutual aid group for people who suffer from diabetes has been meeting for twelve months. It comprises ten people—six women and four men. Membership has been stable for about six months, during which time the participants have formed close and supportive bonds with one another. Two members left within the first six weeks and two joined about six months ago. The purpose of this ongoing open group for people recently diagnosed with adult-onset diabetes is to provide opportunities for members to learn from one another about their condition and to relieve the isolation and anxiety associated with it. Meetings have focused on issues to do with how participants have been managing their health in relation to family and work commitments. The group is led by a social worker, Anne, who set up the group, drawing participants from people who attend the Community Health Centre where she works. Anne's practice has been to interview potential participants to assess their suitability, taking into account their age, compatibility with other participants and interest in using the group for the purpose she has outlined.

As the group has been very stable in terms of membership for a relatively long period of time, Anne is aware that a new member may destabilise the group and be perceived as threatening the closeness and intimacy participants seem to have established. At the same time, she is concerned that the group has almost become a closed group and that people are 'too comfortable'. Her sense is that a new member may offer the opportunity for members to be challenged by an 'outsider' and that this could help them move on more constructively. A patient is referred to her whom she thinks will benefit from group work and will fit in well with the group. She assesses Jill and invites her to join after she has had the opportunity to inform the group of this decision. At the next group meeting, Anne mentions to the group that another person will be joining them.

At first members are rather silent. Then George asks whether the new member is a male or female. After stating that it will be a woman, Anne asks George what difference gender will make to him. This leads to a discussion of the male/female balance in the group and some anxiety is expressed that the men in the group will be outnumbered still further. The importance of a gender balance to this group has not been focused on to any significant degree before. This then leads to talk about the different roles that men and women have played in the group to date and some development of this idea in relation to men and women's different and complimentary experiences of diabetes. Anne recognises that there is both anxiety and some anger emerging in relation to the lack of consultation members feel they have had about the kind of new member they want. The power of the leader to make such decisions then becomes the focus of their anger, and mixed with it there is some resentment that her decision has upset their comfort zone. Towards the end of the meeting, members begin to consider what it will be like to have 'new blood' in the group and how this might be a positive contribution. They also express some empathy towards the new member, recognising that she too has diabetes and that, just as the group has helped them, it will also help Jill. By the time the meeting ends, they are talking with a mixture of excited anticipation and some resignation about her coming—how it will be for Jill joining a group of ten people whom she doesn't know but who are all very familiar with one another.

Jill comes to the next meeting. The majority of members are present at the start but two arrive late and two (a man and a woman) send apologies that they cannot attend. Without prompting from Anne, members introduce themselves by name. Anne suggests that it may be helpful for Jill if people say a bit about themselves and why they are in the group. This provides a useful 'ice breaker' and a good way for participants to take stock of their own progress and expectations of the group. During a silent pause in the latter half of the session, Anne reflects on the anxiety that everyone probably feels at the arrival of a new person, including Jill, and how a new person really changes the group dynamic—not only is there a new member but there is now also a new group. This reflection is taken up by group members and, with some laughter, they recount their doubts and anxieties of the previous week. Jill too talks about her apprehension and how actually meeting the members has allayed her fears—'we've got a lot in common'. There is also some joking about the latecomers and the absentees: whether or not their actions were related to the change in the group's membership.

Discussion

Several issues are highlighted in this example:

• A group worker always needs to prepare the group for the arrival of a new member.
• The idea of an outsider joining a group stirs up thoughts and feelings that may otherwise remain dormant. Anxieties about being outnumbered, about there being 'too many' in the group for

individuals to receive 'enough' attention, and about the power of the leader to take control away from members may emerge. These issues are important. Should they remain unspoken, they may inhibit members' abilities to form more trusting relationships and increase a sense of the group as an unsafe place. Recognising them may be useful in building self-esteem and allowing participants to appraise their own strengths and resources. The introduction of a new member may provide an opportunity for them to be addressed in ways that enable participants to confront and deal with such thoughts and feelings constructively.

- Joining an existing group is not easy. The group worker may use the assessment interview to explore the potential member's anxieties and fears about this, and to offer support and empathy for the risk-taking of the new member.
- New members change the dynamic of a group and, in effect, create a new group. This is where the capacity to 'think group' alerts us to the way in which the group-as-a-whole is impacted upon by change.
- The group worker usually needs to take an active role in ensuring the 'safe passage' of the new person into the group and the group's accommodation of the change involved.

Conflict in the group: Member to member

It is accepted that there will be upsets and we'll work them out. (Bridget)

We're not here to debate . . . it's about listening, about challenging men to change . . . (Chris)

Conflict in the group? It just killed it for me. (Maria)

Most group workers and participants are anxious about the possibility of anger—who will direct it at whom, how it will be manifested, how it will be handled and by whom (see Yalom 1975, pp. 351–58; Doherty et al. 1996; Conyne 1999, Ch. 6).

Example 1

A social action group formed spontaneously in a street in a middle-class suburb. The street was a cul-de-sac and one end abutted a facility for intellectually disabled people. All the residents of the street had enjoyed their quiet environment, children had played safely in the street and, from time to time, street parties had been organised. When news arrived of plans by the institution to open a back gate to allow the street to become a thoroughfare, the residents met to oppose this move. Residents included doctors, lawyers and accountants who had considerable financial resources as well as influential social networks. Various strategies were proposed: establishing a protest within the grounds when families visited; establishing a picket line to prevent any work taking place; appealing to the local government authorities. At meetings, these ideas were canvassed and there was some quite heated disagreement, particularly when the financial costs of these various strategies was considered. A majority-vote decision-making process had been instigated at the beginning and the most favoured strategy (appealing to local government authorities) was adopted. Those who were out-voted were annoyed and initially refused to provide any financial support to the campaign and the group was in danger of fragmenting. However, as the time for action shortened, members agreed to cooperate and contributed to the appeal in order to avoid the fragmentation of the group and the possible failure of the appeal. This action was successful and the institution abandoned its plans. This success mended the rifts that had begun to appear amongst neighbours. However, the group then disbanded and life in the street returned to its previously harmonious level.

Example 2

Another social action group, advocating for families with children with a chronic medical condition, initially began life as a self-help group. As a self-help group, families would meet to socialise and share knowledge and experiences about living with a child disabled by this condition. However, several families began to see that more was needed: they wanted the group to become an advocacy group, taking issues of concern such as health benefits for medication, integration of the children into normal schools and publicity campaigns to address discrimination at the level of policy. The group numbered about 30 people and less than half of them wanted to turn the group into an advocacy group. Significant conflict erupted which seemed to principally target one of the more active members. She experienced angry outbursts at meetings and on the phone. When the dispute reached crisis point with the threatened resignation of this member and several long-term members, a decision was reached by the pro-advocacy supporters to call in an outside consultant to assist them both in resolving the conflict and deciding on where the group could go in the future. The consultant was a social worker known to many group members and had worked in the field for some time. She and the opposing factions met to establish some common ground. The consultant emphasised the group members' strengths and the important achievements the group had so far made. From these discussions, group members decided to take a two-pronged focus, one arm dealing with the socialising aspect of the group and the other with advocacy. The leadership structure of the group was rearranged, with various members taking responsibility for different portfolios—for example, the social contacts, the policy responses, the family education meetings, and so on. With all these separate pathways identified and the common interest of the group members emphasised, the group has continued to take both an active policy development role as well as an inclusive social network-development role.

Conflict in the group: Member to workers

Example

John had joined a long-term psychotherapy group because of his depression and feelings of low self-esteem. He had not been in a therapy group before and had referred himself to try and improve his situation. He seemed to be fitting in well during the first two meetings; however, by his third meeting he had taken a dislike to the leader, Frank. John felt that Frank's comments were attacks on him and he retaliated with criticism such as: 'Why should I listen to you? You're just trying to be smart and show off your superiority . . . all those qualifications just come from books—you don't know anything about real life . . .' Frank responded by accepting that John's criticism came from feelings of low self-esteem and anxiety that he was not accepted in the group. He commented: 'The fact that you see me in this way must make the group a very uncomfortable place for you. You have not been here very long and it was probably a bit of a risky thing deciding to come into the group.'

Other group members responded to this by talking about how anxious they had felt at the beginning and how their anxiety had made them act in certain ways—for example, by being silent or, like John, being angry. John calmed down a little but then turned on the other members and accused them of trying to protect the leader by siding with him. Quite a bit of conflict erupted at this point with various members becoming angry with John. Frank then tried to both acknowledge the anger and to help members look more closely at what was happening: 'John has really got everyone going now and I wonder whether we are all struggling to see how we can deal with his point of view and understand what he wants from us at the same time as making sure that the anger we are all feeling doesn't divide us.'

Discussion

These various scenarios present us with incidents in which group members have been in conflict with one another and/or with the leader. Various solutions were proposed:

- The social action group against the street opening became task-focused, putting disagreements aside in the interests of achieving the principal goal.
- The advocacy group called in an outside consultant to mediate.
- The psychotherapy group relied on the leader to contain the anger and to use it to promote understanding amongst group members.

The kinds of solutions which emerge depend on the kind of group it is, and this in turn determines how the conflict is interpreted (see Benjamin et al. 1997 pp. 186–87; Conyne 1999, Ch. 5, 6 and 7; Forsyth 1999, Ch. 9; Toseland and Rivas 1998, pp. 305–7). For example, conflict was seen as an interference with the 'main game' of the social action group; in the advocacy group it was seen as an element which could either facilitate or derail the group's development (see Mondros and Berman-Rossi 1991 regarding very similar issues in a community development group). In the psychotherapy group, it was seen as an opportunity for all members to explore and to try to understand better the factors that lead to anger and how these affect individuals' emotional lives. Again, the capacity to see how the group-as-a-whole makes sense of a situation draws on the group worker's attention to 'thinking group'.

When conflict occurs in a group (and it does in all groups, whether or not it is recognised), the group worker's task is:

- to try to understand its meaning and impact in relation to the group's purpose and to the group-as-a-whole;
- to contain it so that it does not become a divisive influence. The group worker might do this by:
  - identifying that it is present;

- encouraging members to explore it;
- making rules—for example, outlawing abusive language or physical attack;
- providing the group with a number of ways of handling it— for example, by structuring the meeting so that everyone will be able to speak, suggesting different interpretations of what the conflict might mean, setting up a decision-making structure to resolve the dispute, etc.;
- ensuring that there are adequate opportunities for members to debrief afterwards, whether in the group or individually.

The 'uncooperative' group

... nobody wants to come through that door to see me ... (Chris)

There are a number of settings and purposes which result in groups being established with a 'reluctant' or non-voluntary membership (see Toseland and Rivas 1998, p. 152, 195–97; Shulman 1999, Ch. 11). For example, as we saw in Chapter 2, Chris Laming's group for men who are violent would fall into this category. Some men were referred from the criminal justice system but others had decided to join it themselves as a result of their behaviour and its possible implications in the future. Other settings where groups are set up, such as prisons or accommodation facilities for disabled or elderly people, may include people who are not there under their own volition. To a lesser extent, educational settings which require students to be part of a group in order to take part in experiential learning may be met with some reluctance and a feeling that they are being pressured to join in because of assessment protocols. All these settings create contradictions. Even under the best possible conditions, working in groups may be perceived as intended to enhance participants' freedom to think and act. At the same time, however, the very existence of a group which one is compelled to join contravenes this.

It would be unusual if these conditions of compulsion or the involuntary nature of participation did not have a significant impact. There may be overt signs from members that they are unhappy being in the group, such as angry or threatening outbursts, or more subtle indicators such as being argumentative, criticising the leader and other participants, appearing bored, uninterested or reluctant to take part, or frequently being late in arriving or leaving early. These ways of acting suggest that participants are responding to their situation by becoming resistant and closing off to gaining anything from the group. As Helen pointed out (written communication), voluntary group participants can take direct action and leave the group; those who are involuntary can absent their 'hearts and minds'. Constructive participation becomes the first casualty.

Example

Susan, a final-year social work student, began her placement in a hostel for aged persons. This had not been her first choice for a place-ment but she was determined to make the most of it. However, her initial impression was that many of the residents were equally unhappy to be there. She noticed that new arrivals in particular were occasionally tearful and some of the residents who had been there for longer periods had an air of sadness and resignation about them. Two weeks after beginning her placement, Susan was approached by both nursing staff and several relatives of residents with suggestions that she begin a support group for them. At first Susan thought this would be an excellent idea and began planning various activities that such a group might do. The group's purpose would be to build support and friendships amongst the residents.

Susan decided that she could begin by asking residents what they would like a group to do. However, the first three residents she approached—one newly arrived and the other two having been there for six months—all opposed the idea. 'All I want,' Mr J said, 'is to leave here as soon as I can.' Mrs L agreed: 'I'm not putting down roots here—I've got a lovely home to go back to as soon as I get my strength back.' Mr W hardly waited for Susan to complete her question: 'They'll [the staff] do anything to get us to quiet down and put up with the muck they call food—a support group—no thanks!'

These comments resonated with Susan's own reluctance about being at the hostel. She could see immediately that the proposed group represented the wishes of everyone except those for whom it was intended—yet she also believed that perhaps, if it was carefully designed, it could improve the residents' quality of life. The dilemma she faced was how to construct and offer it in a way which acknowledged the limitations imposed by the setting and still maximised the potential of residents to give and receive emotional support to and from one another.

Discussion

Susan's dilemma is not unusual and, as we have noted, it could equally apply in a number of situations. Depending on the type of group proposed and the population for whom it is intended, there are several ways in which group workers might confront these problems. The group worker might:

- identify and clarify the group's espoused purpose at the outset, so everyone knows what it is. For example, the worker might emphasise the learning opportunity the group provides, or the chance participants have to think about and reflect on what they know, or the potential the group has for relieving isolation and loneliness by connecting with others in similar situations;
- make sure that participants are not being deceived—for example, by ignoring the fact that, in the case of an experiential learning

group, participants are expected to take some risks and may find themselves disclosing things about themselves that would not occur in a 'regular' tutorial;

- be aware of the likely consequences which non-voluntary participation may have—for instance, how participants may be angry or irritated and how participants may act on this rather than talking about it;

- explore these consequences with participants, making them aware that the group worker him/herself is also aware of how they might feel about their participation;

- set clear goals which are able to be achieved despite the constraints of the setting or reason for the group's existence. For example, residents may not be able to make changes to the facility they live in, but they may be able to form closer, more supportive bonds with others through group participation to help them cope better with the problems;

- provide opportunities for participants to set the agenda—for example, have input into the kinds of activities or tasks they want to perform;

- encourage as much autonomy and control within the group as possible—for example, by ensuring that, where decisions are needed, a democratic process is used, or encouraging participants to keep a reflective journal where they can express their own thoughts and ideas about what is happening in the group and chose to share or not share this material;

- be very clear where boundaries lie and ensure that participants are aware of these—for example, that physical or verbal abuse is not tolerated but that talk about such angry or aggressive feelings is welcomed;

- ensure that he or she does not make claims for the group which are beyond what is possible; rather, that the group worker acknowledges the limitations imposed by the setting or the group's purpose.

The silent member

We've all seen several people go through [who were not suited]—
one was destructive to the group, another said practically nothing
...I wish she'd had more time with us ... (Breast Cancer
Therapy Group)

You need skills to deal with dominating or reticent people—
acknowledging what they're saying without putting them down.
(Janet)

People in groups often become resentful of a member who speaks
little, especially in a group which is talk-based, such as a counselling
or psychotherapy group. (For a discussion of different roles in groups,
see Yalom 1975, Ch. 112; Benson 1987; Shulman 1999, Ch. 13.)

Example

Peter had been in a long-term psychotherapy group for several months,
during which time he rarely spoke. He had joined an ongoing group
comprising three men and five women with the espoused purpose of
becoming 'more comfortable' in groups. He was unemployed and,
although he had professional qualifications, showed little interest in
pursuing work, while expressing anger (on the rare occasions when he
spoke) at the difficulties he encountered as an unemployed person. For
the most part, he would arrive late at the group and sit in silence, often
with his eyes closed. His non-verbal presence suggested that he was
angry and depressed. Other members had welcomed him when he
joined but did not press him to talk. From time to time, the leader
would invite him to share his thoughts, especially when a topic was
being discussed that seemed as if it might relate to him; on other
occasions the leader would refer to his silence and attempt to interpret
it in order to bring him into the conversation—for example, 'Peter

might also be angry about this but perhaps feels unsafe to voice his feelings . . .'

After several months, the leader wondered whether it was more helpful to Peter to leave him to initiate talk. Leader-generated attempts to bring him into the conversations did not seem to be helping him join in under his own steam. The leader began to feel irritated with him and noticed that other group members also felt this way. Interestingly, however, some group members felt very warmly towards him, perhaps recognising in his silence something they could identify with. One evening, only four members were present, including Peter. He appeared to be more comfortable with the smaller size of the group and was quite vocal. At this point, the leader was able to raise the issue of safety in talking in a group and Peter and the others explored this in detail, especially as safety seemed to relate to the number of people present. In subsequent meetings, Peter began to initiate more talk and became relatively expansive in discussing some of the pressures and stresses he had experienced in his life.

Discussion

Silence in a talk-based group can create tensions for group leaders and other members alike. Because a person is silent, it is very difficult to know what prevents them speaking and the members and leader may be torn between letting the person 'be' and prompting them to join in. Silent members may sometimes be seen as critical and oppressive and at other times as 'not pulling their weight' and thus as a drain on the group. Neither position is comfortable or helpful to the collective endeavour and therefore this situation needs attending to. In the example provided above, the leader took a role in reaching out to Peter and attempting to help him find a place within the group. The other members did not do so overtly, but indicated by their interest in him whenever he spoke that he was included and considered part of the group. Neither of these strategies was particularly successful and

Peter's silence seemed, in his mind, to relate to anxieties over the number of people in the group. When he had the experience (perhaps even the added pressure) of a small number of people, he was able to risk talking. The positive outcome from this enabled him to begin the process of establishing connections with others and using the group process for the purpose he had desired.

From this example of a silent member, several points are worth noting:

- Silence in a talk-based group requires attention from the group worker: it is clearly an issue for the group-as-a-whole and it needs to be dealt with carefully.
- Other group members will be trying to make sense of the silent member's silence themselves; sometimes silence may be perceived as oppressive and threatening and a source of discomfort. The silent member is likely to become the target of other members' anxieties and hostilities.
- The group worker needs to take care not to over-interpret what the member's silence means but rather to use comments which are sufficiently open-ended and encouraging in order to reduce the member's anxiety at the same time as supporting the member to risk talking.

The dominating member

One of the consumers was very disturbed by his experience, so he took over. It was very hard to contain him in the group. (Janet)

People can dominate groups in all sorts of ways, including through their silence or constant absence. Members sometimes become angry or feel alienated by one member's seeming to take over or even to be, too often, the focus of the group's attention. However, people who are most often seen to dominate a group tend to be those who are extremely talkative.

Example

Clare was such a person in a psychoeducational group for women who were carers of a person with a serious mental illness. The group had been meeting for several weeks, focused around the sharing of ideas about how best to care for oneself despite the enormous demands the caring role exerted. Two outside speakers had already addressed the group and a video on the topic was screened. Clare's story had much in common with others in the group and for several meetings they listened with interest to her account of managing her life. However, by about the fourth week, other members had begun to withdraw into silence, showing signs of boredom and irritation. By about the sixth meeting, several members were absent but Clare continued to talk in increasing detail about the issues of importance to her. The group leader played around with several possible ways of dealing with this situation. She decided that she had a number of choices:

- to ignore the situation and allow Clare to keep talking and watch the group disintegrate;
- to meet with Clare on her own outside the group and tell her to allow more space for others to talk;
- to suggest privately to Clare that her problems and issues would be more appropriately dealt with in individual counselling and to suggest she leave the group;
- to invite other members to challenge Clare by, for example, asking them how they felt about her dominating talk;
- to work with Clare in the group to try to discover what fears, anxieties or other emotions prompted her to talk excessively. This may assist Clare in developing some insight into the causes of her behaviour and the possibly alienating consequences they had for her by driving away any support she may have needed. By doing this in the group, others could learn from this and at the same time offer Clare support in changing her behaviour;

- to draw from Clare's stories themes and ideas which others might share and invite them to contribute their reflections;
- to interrupt Clare and instigate a 'ten minutes each' rule for participants to talk.

Discussion

Clare's situation is not an uncommon one in many groups. The group leader, 'thinking group' and seeing what was happening in the group-as-a-whole, had decided that her dominating behaviour was having a damaging effect on the group and was preventing the group from developing beyond its initial stage. Having made that interpretation, the leader then considered various ways of 'saving' both the group and Clare from a destructive turn of events. The leader's identification of possible action strategies indicated that she was attempting to balance both the needs of individuals with those of the collective. There are always several possible ways of handling a situation and in this example the leader's choice of which one (or ones) to adopt may have depended on:

- the purpose of the group. A psychoeducational group usually tries to incorporate both experiential and didactic input following a pre-determined schedule. The leader will need to judge to what extent Clare's behaviour will prevent the group's purpose being satisfactorily achieved;
- the number of sessions the group is scheduled to run—in other words, how much time is available to meet the needs of the members and thus how much urgency there is for dealing with Clare's behaviour. A short-term group of about twelve sessions has relatively little time available, so that the leader may decide to act more directly than would be the case in an open, long-term group;
- the way in which the group is structured—that is, what kind of role the leader has assumed. This might determine who should

challenge Clare, whether other participants should be supported to do so, or whether the leader herself should act independently;
• the leader's theoretical position. For example, if the leader identifies the group as a system requiring some kind of maintenance or repair, or if the leader is working from a position which views the group as a site for meaning-construction, this will affect which strategy will be adopted. Other theoretical perspectives might generate other strategies.

A member's decision to leave

. . . [a limitation of the group] is . . . living with the awareness of [a participant's] unfinished issues. In the counselling session where it's just you and her you get a much better chance to work through an issue. In a group the issue can get chopped off, so you go away yourself not knowing how she was, being left with that— this is a cost . . . (Heather)

. . . [you need] clarity of purpose . . . and not to be afraid to explore and respectfully initiate a group process—it develops . . . (Chris)

Example

Joan had been a member of a psychoanalytically oriented psychotherapy group since it began. She joined the group after discussions with her psychotherapist who co-leads the group. Joan was in her mid-40s. She was a physiotherapist but had been unable to work in her profession since experiencing severe depression about twelve months before joining the group. Her purpose in joining the group was to engage with others in order to break out of her isolation and to receive support and assistance in finding ways of counteracting her depression. On joining the group, Joan played an important role in reaching out to others and offering them warmth and sympathy, sometimes with the giving of advice. She remained rather reticent about her own situation but did begin to become more trusting as time went on, revealing her homosexuality and, at one point, telling them that she was undergoing ECT (shock treatment). Her tendency to give advice was at times challenged by other members, which she found difficult to deal with. However, it was still a surprise to other participants that, after eighteen months in the group, she came to a session and revealed her intention to leave. Her reasons were: 'Nothing has changed . . . I've been in this group all this time and I haven't been able to really talk about myself . . . so now I want to leave . . .'

Other members were uncertain how to react. They wanted her to stay and felt that she had achieved changes—for example, that she was now working again as a physiotherapist. They pointed out to her that, as she had recognised her lack of ability to confide in the group, this could now provide a reason to go on and also an agenda for work. At the same time, no one wanted to force her to stay. As per the agreement all members made on entering the group, Joan wanted to use several sessions to discuss her decision before she actually left. During these sessions, members helped Joan explore the reasons prompting her decision. However, Joan remained firm in her decision and left the group. This incident was confronting for all members. Joan had been a consistent and original member of the group. Her decision caused them to reassess their own participation, what they were getting from the group, and the extent to which their own goals were being achieved. This was unsettling for many and a sense of doubt and self-questioning became evident. Joan was well liked by most of them but had been in conflict with one member, Bob. Bob admitted he was pleased she was going and this, in turn, created tensions amongst members—those who felt he was being cruel and insensitive and those who were pleased about his honesty. This tension was uncomfortable and people became irritable with each other. There was a feeling that the co-leaders should 'do something' to relieve the tension, that they were in some sense responsible for Joan's decision through their inactivity and apparent failure to create a group that could meet members' needs.

Discussion

Several issues are relevant here:

*   the impact Joan's decision had on all members;
*   the possibility that one member's decision to leave can undermine the stability of the group and perhaps threaten its continuity;
*   the dilemma members felt between wanting to advocate for Joan's freedom to chose to stay or leave, and the wish to make her stay as it became apparent that her decision to leave may not be in her best interests—that is, she was seen as leaving just at the point when her insight into what she wanted and needed had been clarified, shared with the group, and could now be addressed by the group;
*   the tendency to 'turn against' the co-leaders as having failed the group.

From the point of view of the co-leaders, this incident reinforced:

*   the necessity of ensuring that there is adequate time available for such an important issue as leaving to be discussed thoroughly, precisely because it does have an impact on all group members;
*   the importance of advising members, before they join, that decisions to leave must be addressed *inside* the group and *several sessions* in advance of the departure;
*   the need to enable all members to think about their own situation in relation to the departing member and to use this time as an occasion for reassessing their own situation;
*   that such a decision will generate anger and disappointment and that this may be directed towards the leaders. The leaders need to handle this by acknowledging members' feelings and helping

them to recognise that some anger may target the leaving person but be deflected on to the leaders, demonstrating anxiety that they too might desert the group. It is important for the leaders to reinforce their commitment to the group, and belief in the value and sustainability of the group even when members leave;

* the autonomy of group members to decide for themselves whether to stay or leave, and the continuing availability of the group should they want to return.

The final meeting of a group

Being a time-limited group can be limiting . . . maybe we could take some of the urgency out of it if we gave more than one session to a topic. (Heather)

. . . replicating in here what you then go and do out there . . . (Lou)

Time-limited groups, by definition, conclude by a certain date and time. Members will know in advance that the group will have, for example, ten meetings. However, even if they are aware that the group is to finish, this event may still bring up difficult issues for participants.

Example

A psychoeducational group for parents of people recently diagnosed with schizophrenia has been organised with twelve meetings. The purpose of this group is to provide both educational input about what is known about the possible causes of schizophrenia, the likely behavioural problems that may occur, and suggestions for how parents might cope. There are five couples attending the group so far. By week ten, participants are in agreement that it has been an extremely positive experience. Attendance has been good and participants have found the didactic input helpful and informative. Discussion has been lively and a range of emotions—sadness, grief, humour—have been expressed. All couples appear to have bonded well together and to have recognised that there is considerable common ground amongst them. As the final meeting draws near, the group leader initiates discussion about how members have experienced the group and what will happen to them, as a group, when the program ends. In reflecting on the group experience, participants offer positive feedback about what they have gained from it—principally the opportunity to meet others confronting the same issues and the sense of not being alone. They realise that the absence of the group will be a loss and suggestions are put forward as to how it might be possible for the participants to continue to meet privately once the group ends. The group leader is supportive of this and makes suggestions about available meeting space at a nearby community health centre.

Discussion

Several points are relevant here:

* The importance of the ending of a group for members, and for the group-as-a-whole, cannot be under-estimated, and there is a need for the group worker to make opportunities for members to discuss this, while ensuring that the date of the ending of the group is remembered.
* Endings are sometimes experienced as emotionally painful for participants. Endings may evoke other losses, such as deaths or abandonment. The leader needs to be attuned to the kinds of reactions the ending may bring up—for example, anger and resentment, sadness, silence—and deal with these by acknowledging them, providing time to explore them, and emphasising the strengths members have and the resources available to them, both emotionally and materially.

- The kind of group it is, is very relevant. A psychoeducational group is time-limited and its purpose (often) is to provide participants with resources of knowledge, information and support. In this group, the members themselves have become an important resource to one another. The group worker recognises this and facilitates the group continuing on, with members providing the necessary resources themselves.
- In this example, only one aspect of the group is terminated: it continues on in another form, perhaps as a self-help group.
- Other types of groups may end without any further follow-on— for example, an inpatient support group, in a rehabilitation setting. In this kind of group, the group worker will act differently, ensuring that the ending concludes the work the group has done together. This might mean, for example, that the leader uses the final sessions to assist members to assess the gains they have made over the life of the group, where they want to go in the future, and what resources they may have to access in order to do this (see Shulman 1999, Ch. 15; Toseland and Rivas 1998, Ch. 14).

Summary

In this chapter we have explored a number of important moments or critical issues in the life of groups which can present challenges to group workers. Examples illustrating these moments in a number of different kinds of groups established with varying purposes were provided. Although, as we have described, the significance of these issues will be understood differently depending on the group's purpose, the type of group it is and the theoretical perspective of the group worker, it is apparent in the examples provided that there are also elements which are common to all groups. All group workers need to think and act strategically and be aware that there are always choices to be made about how best to work with a particular group facing particular issues.

10

DOING 'GOOD' GROUP WORK:
'outward looking and moving On'

What is a 'good' group?

A group that's really important to its members . . . (Maria)

It gives you proof of progress, validates skills, confidence, self-esteem . . . (Bridget)

A group where there's good bonding and caring and support—compassion . . . (Breast Cancer Therapy Group)

A mutual support and a mutual challenge . . . (Chris)

[The group gives] opportunities to see themselves reflected back by the group—[this] gives them strength. (Heather)

These comments by group leaders and participants highlight some of the elements they identify as central to a 'good' group—participants' sense of ownership of the group, the support and challenge the group provides, the possibilities groups hold for increasing self-understanding. These comments also indicate just how difficult it is to pinpoint those factors which seem to be responsible for the benefits groups bring to participants and leaders. And they highlight the perceived and sometimes actual gap between research and group work practice (Anderson 1987). Heather speaks for many of us when she says: 'I'm not clear what factors make groups work.'

Researchers and academics have likewise struggled to develop and test outcome criteria. For example, Schoenholtz-Reed (1996, p. 223) comments that, while clinical experience shows that women-only groups are effective, there is no research that consistently demonstrates this. Bloch and Aveline (1996, pp. 93–98) propose that there are a number of factors which they consider provide the therapeutic value of group psychotherapy. These share ground with Yalom's (1975) 'curative factors', discussed in Chapter 3.

In Bloch and Aveline's view, a 'good' group is cohesive and accepting, enabling participants to offer and accept feedback and comment which can extend self-understanding; itself a key goal of recapitulation and restitution groups in particular. Finding others who have similar experiences in the group strengthens the individual's sense of being engaged in a shared endeavour, which allows the emergence of a sense of hope that change is possible and life can be different. Group participants become willing to help one another, at times offering guidance and demonstrating altruism and sensitivity. Simultaneously, they learn from one another through listening and observing. Such a process can facilitate self-disclosure, and the emotional release that comes with this may prompt greater self-understanding. Support and rehabilitation groups and growth and education groups, as we saw earlier (Chapter 7), place particular emphasis on the value of support and learning and evidence of these elements emerging would be highly significant in estimating the 'goodness' of such groups.

Interestingly, as we can see from the quotations at the beginning of this chapter, the factors identified by Bloch and Aveline (1996)

support the anecdotal and experiential evidence sought, and sometimes found, by participants and group leaders. They refer particularly
to issues of group process (see Chapter 8) and, as such, refer
principally to the less tangible but often especially fulfilling aspects of
group participation. For task and action groups, the successful
achievement of the group's target—for example, the retention of a
medical centre or the abandonment of plans to build a freeway—are
readily available measures of an effective group.

Nevertheless, it is a very important part of working with groups
to be able to think about how practice can be improved, about what
'works' and what 'doesn't work', and about how 'good' practice can
become 'better' practice. This is not an easy task, especially if we
consider the particular problematics that researchers face in studying
groups.

The most striking characteristic of all groups is their complexity—the multiple 'layers' of intersecting interaction and fluid
meanings which occur over time, and within a context, and which all
go into making the experience and the process of a group. Everyone
in a group becomes both participant and observer; power shifts as
meanings are constructed, negotiated, challenged or allowed to
prevail. Such a turbulent and transient phenomenon poses considerable problems for those who wish to research groups and, perhaps to
an extent, explains the relatively limited amount of available research
(Rose and Feldman 1987; Tindale et al. 1998). However, every group
can also be thought of as an ongoing process of research-in-action—
indeed, groups owe their vitality and energy to the fact that they are
continually researching themselves. As Long (1992, p. 78) points out,
groups 'constantly interact with the results of their own observations'.
In fact, they can be thought of as exemplifying participatory action
research (McTaggart 1993; Wadsworth 1997), characterised by a cycle
of action, reflection on that action, and further action. This is the case
regardless of the type of group or the time-frame it has adopted.
A social action or task group may take concrete action to achieve its

goals—for example, setting up a drop-in centre for homeless people—but this will be an outcome of a process of debate and collaboration in which original goals and purposes are revisited and reviewed. A psychotherapy group may assist a participant to think through an important decision, but in the process others will be engaged in reviewing their own ways of thinking and acting, weighing up whether or not the group is able to help them. Considering groups to be sites of research-in-action also alerts us to what Long (1992, p. 79) refers to as a 'data problem'. Because the meanings of actions and processes within the group are not self-evident, but rather emerge through the exchanges and interactions taking place amongst participants, we need to understand the context (both internal and external to the group) and how it is being constructed and interpreted in the minds of participants. This is challenging.

While these particular problematics confront anyone wanting to evaluate and research groups, they do not mean that the task is impossible. A set of suggested guidelines to finding out how well a group is working and how it might work better are discussed below. These are formulated with group workers as 'insider' researchers in mind—that is, towards those who are participants in groups, whether as designated leaders or as members who want to know how best to capture what is happening in the group. From this basis, decisions about how to 'go on' in shaping the group towards achieving its purposes can be instigated. In keeping with our earlier discussion of the central importance of group workers 'thinking group'—that is, working from the perspective of the group-as-a-whole—these guidelines proceed from a view, shared by Glisson (1987, p. 15), that the focus must be on the *group* as the unit of attention and analysis rather than on individuals. While we may identify changes that individuals achieve, what these mean and how they were arrived at refer specifically to the nature and interpretation made of the experience of working together. Clearly, then, individuals working together must be studied as such, from the viewpoint that there is some kind of relationship between individuals in a group which may account for the changes we observe or assert have occurred for individuals.

Guidelines for studying the group's progress

This book has been organised according to five main components of groups: purpose, theory, leading, form and structure, and time. Each of these components can now be considered as a 'window' through which we can view and study the group's progress. As we have argued throughout, each of these elements is closely interwoven with the others. The purpose the group adopts reflects the way in which a particular issue or event has been problematised. In turn, how the issue or event is problematised indicates the theoretical basis under-pinning the group's formation, who will be in it, whether it will be time-unlimited or time-limited, open or closed. The way in which the group worker works will emerge from the theoretical frame adopted which will then influence the degree and extent of reciprocity in relationships within the group. The kind of 'life' the group takes on will refer to the time-scale available for participants to achieve their individual and collective goals. It will also refer to the particular resources which participants, including the leader, bring to their collective work: their knowledge, experience, structural positioning, and capacity to manage the complexity and fluidity of relationships which the phenomenon of the group unleashes.

As a way of 'looking through' these five 'windows' on to the group, the following guidelines—or questions to signpost our inquiries—may be useful.

Purpose

- Where did the idea for this group come from? Whose idea was it?
- What is the group's espoused purpose or purposes?

- Does everyone in the group share the same understanding of the purpose(s)?
- Have the purpose(s) changed?

Theory

- What theoretical perspective(s) best capture the underlying conceptualisation of this group?
- What 'evidence' is there that this is the prevailing theoretical perspective—for example, in the way the group's purpose has been formulated, or the way in which the group came into existence?

Leading

- Is there a designated leader or facilitator? Co-leaders? Have 'internal leaders' emerged?
- How much sharing of the tasks of leading or influencing the group's purposes is apparent? For example, who does what and when?

Form and structure

- What type of group is this? For example, is it open or closed? Time-limited or time-unlimited?
- Who is in it? For example, what ages, genders, abilities, sexuality, ethnicity and class characterise participants?
- What are the 'pathways' into the group? For example, are people recruited or do they join voluntarily?
- What activities take place? Are they planned or spontaneous? Why have these activities been chosen?
- Where does the group meet? What physical arrangements have been made?

Time

- What time-frame has been adopted or established?
- What changes are occurring over time? For example, have participants begun to bond with one another? Are people staying? Has anyone left before they have had an opportunity to become involved? Did people leave because they were in some way unhappy with what was happening?
- Do people talk and listen to one another? Does anyone dominate the talk? Is anyone silent for long periods?
- How would you characterise the climate of the group? For example, is it warm and comfortable, tension-filled, hostile?
- Is there a feeling of cohesion—that the group has begun to matter to participants? Are there signs of trust emerging? What form has conflict taken? How and by whom was it managed?
- Are the group's purposes, both espoused and emergent, being achieved? In what ways? What 'evidence' is there? For example, do participants talk of dealing more effectively with their everyday problems in living? Has the group achieved change in an issue or problem being targeted, such as being consulted by policy-makers?
- Did people in the group behave differently towards one another as time elapsed? For example, can some people be challenged and use this to help them think about themselves rather than becoming defensive? Has the designated leader relinquished some control of the process by, for example, encouraging others to express support for their fellow participants?

Monitoring the group's progress

These guidelines are designed to draw our attention to the observable signs indicating the extent and ways in which the group is working. Of course, the questions we ask of the group in this way also reflect our approach to group work, the particular issues we identify as significant. Importantly, how we pose, interpret and make sense of them will depend on the theoretical and knowledge base that informs our practice. Getting at this dimension of understanding what is happening in a group suggests we may need additional strategies. Adopting one or all (or some additional) strategies, as discussed below, is a key aspect in strengthening our capacity to 'think group'— to know how to 'go on' as group workers and to acquire further capabilities in reflecting on our practice in working with a group. We will explore two complementary ways of monitoring the group's and our own work: recording and reflection.

Recording

In a review and analysis of extant research on groups, Tindale et al. (1998, p. 3) note that the practice of group work extends across many different domains. However, there has been fragmentation and little sharing of ideas and methods across disciplines, although considerable attention has been given to the study of how groups work in a variety of settings. In their overview of research, the authors note that despite this fragmentation, there are several general themes which have received attention from group researchers. These include: leadership; the educational role of groups, not only for training purposes but as a medium for people understanding better and learning more about the conditions of their lives; interdependence—as a defining feature of groups; time and the dynamic nature of groups over time; and group myths—what people believe about groups and the extent to which these beliefs are borne out by research findings. Wright and Gould (1996, pp. 333–50) similarly review the existing research 'by small-group process researchers on the variables of gender composition of the group, the impact of the leader's gender, and the gender of the group member'. While findings within these research areas are important to incorporate into group work practice, it is beyond the purpose of this book to suggest that workers engage in comprehensive research or evaluation programs. Rather, our focus here is on the ways in which group workers can understand and enhance their own practice.

Sullivan (1995, p. 15) notes that there is 'a wealth of data . . . lying available in the written recordings of every group practitioner' awaiting analysis in order to generate theory for practice. What to observe and record and how to do so is, of course, an important decision (see Chapter 6). Bradford (1961, pp. 75–80) describes various techniques for recording in groups. For example, group workers might note who talks to whom, the kind of contributions participants make (for example, offering advice, disagreeing, asking opinions, etc.), and what happens in regard to the climate in the group (for example, competitive, support-ive), the quality and quantity of work accomplished, the leader's behaviour (for example, dominating the group, encouraging communi-cation), and the extent of participation (for example, whether many or few participated, whether members were united or divided). Long (1992, p. 77) similarly reviews the variety of methods through which it is possible to study small groups. These methods are readily available—in fact, they are intrinsic to the practice of group work. They include participant observation and interviewing.

In order to see what kind of observations can be recorded, an example is presented below. These are process notes made by the co-leaders of a long-term open mutual support group for women suffering a life-threatening illness. There are ten women in the group and two female co-leaders. The group's purpose is to provide support, opportunities to express feelings, and the possibility for developing social and supportive networks which operate outside the meeting times. The group meets for one and a quarter hours weekly and has been ongoing for several months. There are seven women present and the two co-leaders. These notes refer to a segment of the group meeting occurring in the first half hour. Notes in italics refer to the co-leaders' interpretations of the non-verbal communications in the group, and the group atmosphere or climate.

What happened	Co-leaders

Helen: I've had a bad week—had a blood test and passed out—my veins have just gone. Then the doctor suggested further tests—I'm just so anxious.

Yvette: You shouldn't read things into it.

Helen: But I can't help it—all those tests are just so awful.

(Everyone is attending very closely to what Helen is saying. There is a sense of rising anxiety and distress.)

> The treatment is worse than the illness.

Helen: we just put up with so much. It's ongoing for the rest of your life.

(Expression of strong feelings of anguish and frustration.)

Pat: but we've got a life.

Yvette: there's always people worse off.

Helen: who is worse off than me? *(Some laughter and some competitive sparring between Yvette and Helen.)* You do laugh about it, but underneath there is some despair and you don't always feel like laughing.

Pat: I get sick of being brave.

Helen: I even began to feel sorry for the doctor!

(Laughter and sense of cameraderie as people recognise themselves in one another.)

> I wonder if you picked up some of the doctor's anxiety?

Helen: maybe so—I didn't use to be anxious.

(Various comments about going to a pathology expert rather than a General Practitioner because of their expertise.)

(Sense of knowing what others have been through—wanting to help with ideas and advice.)

What happened	Co-leaders
	I'm really struck by how we all experience pain in such individual ways—we want to share that but then we worry about upsetting others.

Pat: My daughters ask me 'what are you hiding from us?'
Yvette: My father's the same. He says 'tell us the truth now'.
(Feelings of relief in expressing anxieties and talking about worries on behalf of others.)

These notes provide us with a considerable amount of descriptive information, but the question of what to do with it—how to analyse and use it—is clearly very important. In regard to the above example, the co-leaders might do some of the following:

- They could draw out the themes or recurring ideas that emerged in the meeting.
- They might explore the appropriateness of their interventions— for example, what happened when they commented? Did the discussion develop in a useful direction or did the interventions seem to inhibit what people subsequently said?
- They could also explore what did not happen, or what was not said—what gaps or inconsistencies are evident which might indicate anger or anxiety or fear that was not noticed at the time.
- Given that this group has been meeting for some time, it would be possible to compare the notes from this session with earlier sessions. What is being talked about today? Who is contributing? Who seems to be silent? What themes or emotions prevail across several sessions?
- In relation to this context—that of an ongoing group—they could look at what change or movement or recycling can be observed. What does this tell us about how the group is impacting on

participants and how participants are impacting on the group?
• They could examine what evidence there is that the group's purposes are being achieved.

Getzch (1988, pp. 115–28) offers a similar strategy which draws on Schon's (1983) conceptualisation of reflection-in-action. Group workers are advised to keep a 'record of service', which is a log or process record of what takes place in the group, including both verbal and non-verbal events. The log is reviewed by the group worker who notes particular problems he or she experiences, or problems that the group-as-a-whole may have experienced. The skills the leader used at various points are identified, as well as those interventions which were seen as unhelpful or which could have been done differently. It is of central importance in this process that the group worker, usually during a teaching or supervisory session, engages their imagination through empathy and reflection to try to grasp how particular problems or experiences may have been experienced by group participants. From this process, Getzch (1988) suggests that group workers will be assisted in thinking in new ways about their skills and their practice. This is reminiscent of our earlier discussion on 'thinking group' in Chapter 6. Getzch (1988, p. 127) notes:

In order to solve problems we not only work with theory and concepts, but with the metaphors or our cumulative or summative experiences in groups and with images stored within our brains that elicit the feelings and tone of our present experiences.

Making these insights available for reflection and action comes from using the 'record of service' as a springboard to innovative ways of 'thinking group'.

Sullivan (1995; see also Long 1992, p. 77) provides an account of her work in analysing similarly derived qualitative data from a number of group meetings. Drawing on data analysis methods frequently used in qualitative research, Sullivan demonstrates the process of classify-ing, categorising and analysing these data in ways which get beyond the self-evident and yet are interpreted and made meaningful within the context in which the data emerged.

While our interest here is in suggesting ideas and relatively simple strategies for monitoring the processes within a group, clearly there is considerable room for developing and using much more complicated and in-depth quantitative and qualitative methods (see, for example, Anderson 1987; Long 1992; Tindale et al. 1998). As Papell (1997, p. 13) has commented, there is substantial scope to develop the knowledge and capabilities of group workers' practice as a first priority in 'helping the group to grow'.

Reflection

Reflection on practice in any domain is central to developing our capac-ities and knowledge base. A number of the methods noted above for recording group data also rely on strategies for making sense of that data—for example, Getzsch's 'record of service' and Sullivan's use of qualitative methods for content analysis. However, three other methods are essential for all group workers, whether beginning or experienced: feedback from the group; feedback from co-leaders; and supervision.

As we described earlier, the group can be thought of as synonymous with the cycles ascribed to participatory action research—action, reflec-tion on action, further action. Consciously shaping the group process to do this, or sharpening one's observational and listening skills, provides ready access to feedback about where the process is heading and how and to what extent it is achieving the group's purpose. Some group workers like to structure this more closely by, for example, requesting participants to complete feedback forms after each meeting. What is very important, however, is to ensure that this feedback is shared with the group, bearing in mind that it is the collective work of the group rather than individual commentaries that provides the 'raw material' the group works with.

Co-leadership, as discussed in Chapter 4, can be another rich source of knowing how one is working. It is important to make time available before and after each session to plan and to share perceptions and differing insights into what happened in the session (Kahn 1996; Corey 2000, pp. 55–62). This is an excellent way of learning about and developing one's capabilities and thinking.

Opportunities for supervision from more experienced group workers need to be found. This could take the form of one-to-one work or could be in a group with other group workers. There are many different models of supervision, most varying in relation to the particular theoretical frame the group works within. The most important role supervision can fulfil is to assist the practitioner in the task of integrating theoretical and practice knowledge or, as Thompson (2000, p. 180) emphasises 'the value of using theory to guide practice and practice to test theory . . . translating the adventure of theory into a practical realm'. Making and taking opportunities to reflect and to develop one's capabilities is vital to 'keeping afloat'—and keeping ahead—in practice that is enormously complex and uncertain. It underscores the fact that the group worker practitioner-in-action is also (potentially at least) a group worker theoretician-in-action.

Summary

In this chapter, a number of ways of assessing whether or not a group is working well in achieving its purposes have been outlined, bearing in mind the difficulty this poses by virtue of a group's fluidity and complexity. The importance of having a framework for viewing the elements which comprise the group's progress and processes was outlined. The usefulness of recording the group's work as it happens and of finding opportunities to receive supervision were suggested as helpful in developing all group workers' abilities to reflect and enhance their practice.

EPILOGUE

Throughout this book, the thoughts and ideas of group 'insiders'—group workers and participants—have accompanied our progress, emphasising and enlivening issues and concepts central to group work practice. Their comments have given us glimpses of the variety and challenge which characterise group work; often, too, their words have hinted at concepts and experiences which deserve more detailed and analytic attention beyond the scope of this book. So it seems fitting to conclude this book with some final comments from these group insiders that highlight what is both unique and shared about working with and in groups.

> You may not have the same political persuasion, you may be from all walks of life but that's one thing that keeps us together, that we have a common purpose. It's pretty unique. (Maria)

> What a small group like this does is that it acts as a kind of midway point between the self and an intimate relationship ... having a place where intimacy can be expressed which is outside

a two-person relationship means you also become less dependent on that relationship . . . you can have intimacy needs met through a group. (Bob)

[We don't really know] how people are experiencing [the group]. We can only know that people come back and are incredibly positive about that experience. (Lou)

These men are struggling and that has to be respected . . . [the group] is about building up the good stuff. (Chris)

[It's] a very enjoyable group to work with because often they are new couples with a high commitment to making their relationship and their family work . . . this is a new beginning. (Robyn)

There's a sharing among the membership—it's got a life of its own. (Cynthia)

I've seen a number of people come and go from this group and they've obviously benefitted from being part of it. They come in uncertain about lots of things about themselves and become more confident in their demeanor, and say things which indicate that they've got it together a bit better than they had previously. For myself I can certainly say it's helped me understand things about myself that I had not understood before. (Bernard)

We also met a whole stack of people that we maybe [had] only known to walk past in the street. So it's a good way to build connections. (Helen)

You learn a great deal from everybody else's experiences and treatments and you get more information about treatment and drugs than the doctors even give you. If we get articles we bring them in and share them around—we share everything around! (Breast Cancer Therapy Group)

You've got to be a bit nuts to do it! (Maria)

There's a potential for things to happen more than in the one-to-one—we can have a lot of fun . . . (Heather)

REFERENCES

Adams, M.V. 1997 'Metaphors in psychoanalytic theory and therapy', *Clinical Social Work Journal*, Vol. 25, No. 1, Spring, pp. 27–39

Anderson, J.D. 1987 'Integrating research and practice in social work with groups', in *Research in Social Groupwork*, S.D. Rose and R.A. Feldman eds, Haworth Press, New York

Anthony, E.J. 1971 'The history of group psychotherapy', in *Comprehensive Group Psychotherapy*, H. Kaplan and B. Saddock eds, Williams & Wilkins, Baltimore

Arminen, I. 1998 'Sharing experiences: Doing therapy with the help of mutual references in the meetings of Alcohlics Anonymous', *The Sociological Quarterly*, Vol. 39, No. 3, pp. 491–513

Barthes, R. 1989 *The Rustle of Language*, University of California Press, Berkeley

Baum, F., Palmer, C., Modra, C., Murray, L. and Bush, R. 2000 'Families, social capital and health', in *Social Capital and Public Policy in Australia*, I. Winter ed., Australian Institute of Family Studies, Melbourne

Beck, U. 1986 *Risk Society: Towards a New Modernity*, Sage, London

Benjamin, J., Bessant, J. and Watts, R. 1997 *Making Groups Work*, Allen & Unwin, Sydney

Benson, J. 1987 *Working More Creatively with Groups*, Routledge, London

Berger, R. 1996 'A comparative analysis of different methods of teaching group work', *Social Work with Groups*, Vol. 19, No. 1, pp. 79–89

Berman-Rossi, T. 1992 'Empowering groups through understanding stages of group development', *Social Work With Groups*, Vol. 15, Nos 2/3, pp. 239–55

Bernardez, T. 1996 'Conflicts with anger and power in women's groups', in *Women and Group Psychotherapy: Theory and practice*, B. DeChant ed., Guilford Press, New York

Bloch, S. and Aveline, M. 1996 'Group psychotherapy', in *An Introduction to the Psychotherapies*, S. Bloch ed., Oxford University Press, New York

Bradford, L. ed. 1961 *Group Development*, National Training Laboratories, Washington, DC

Brower, A.M. 1996 'Group development as constructed social reality revisited: The constructivism of small groups', *Families in Society*, Vol. 77, No. 6, pp. 336–44

Brown, A. 1989 *Groupwork*, 2nd edn, Gower, Aldershot

——1992 *Groupwork*, 3rd edn, Gower, Aldershot

Brown, P.A. and Dickey, C. 1992 'Critical reflection in groups with abused women', *Affilia*, Vol. 16, No. 2, pp. 159–79

Burkhardt, Steve 1982 *The Other Side of Organizing*, Schenkman, Cambridge, MA

Butler, S. and Wintram, C. 1995 *Feminist Groupwork*, Sage, London

Byrt, W.J. 1978 *Leaders and Leadership*, Sun Books, Melbourne

Capra, F. 1988 *Uncommon Wisdom*, Rider, Melbourne

Cohn, B.R. 1996 'Narcissism in women in groups: The emerging female self' in *Women and Group Psychotherapy: Theory and practice*, DeChant, B. ed, Guildford Press, New York

Conyne, R.K. 1999 *Failures in Group Work: How we can learn from our mistakes*, Sage, Thousand Oaks, CA

Corey, G. 2000 *Theory and Practice of Group Counselling*, 5th edn, Brooks/Cole, Stamford

Corradi-Fiumara, G. 1990 *The Other Side of Language: A philosophy of listening*, Routledge, London

Cox, E. and Caldwell, P. 2000 'Making policy social', in *Social Capital and Public Policy in Australia*, I. Winter ed., Australian Institute of Family Studies, Melbourne

Croker, C. 1977 'The social functions of rhetorical forms', in *The Social Use of Metaphor*, D. Sapir and C. Croke eds, University of Pennsylvania Press, Philadelphia

Crotty, M. 1998 *The Foundations of Social Research*, Allen & Unwin, Sydney

Davis, R.D. and Jansen, G.G. 1998 'Making meaning of Alcoholics Anonymous for social workers: Myths, metaphors and realities', *Social Work*, Vol. 43, No. 2, pp. 169–82

Dean, R.G. 1993 'Constructivism: An approach to clinical practice', *Smith College Studies in Social Work*, Vol. 63, No. 2, pp. 127–46

Dean, R.G. 1998 'A narrative approach to groups', *Clinical Social Work Journal*, Vol. 26, No. 1, Spring, pp. 23–37

DeChant, B. ed. 1996 *Women and Group Psychotherapy: Theory and practice*, Guilford Press, New York

Doherty, P., Moses, L.N. and Perlow, J. 1996 'Competition in women: From prohibition to triumph', in *Women and Group Psychotherapy: Theory and practice*, B. DeChant ed., Guilford Press, New York

Douglas, T. 1993 *A Theory of Groupwork Practice*, Macmillan, London

——2000 *Basic Groupwork*, 2nd edn, Routledge, London

Dowds, M.W. 1996 'Paranoia in an ethnically diverse population: The role of group work', *Social Work with Groups*, Vol. 19, No. 1, pp. 67–77

Ebenstein, H. 1998 'Single-session groups: Issues for social workers', *Social Work with Groups*, Vol. 21, Nos 1/2, pp. 49–60

Ezzy, D. 1998 'Theorizing narrative identity: Symbolic interactionism and hermeneutics', *The Sociological Quarterly*, Vol. 39, No. 2, pp. 239–52

Flaherty, M. 1999 *A Watched Pot: How we experience time*, New York University Press, New York

Flannery, K., Irwin, J. and Lopez, A. 2000 'Connection and cultural difference: Women, groupwork and surviving domestic violence', *Women Against Violence*, No. 9, pp. 33–40

Fook, J. 1993 *Radical Casework: A theory for practice*, Allen & Unwin, Sydney

Fook, J. 1999 'Critical reflectivity in education and practice', in *Transforming Social Work Practice: Postmodern critical perspectives*, B. Pease and J. Fook eds, Routledge, London

Forsyth, D.R. 1999 *Group Dynamics*, 3rd edn, Wadsworth, Belmont

Friedman, L. 1999 *The Horizontal Society*, Yale University Press, New Haven, Connecticut

Garland, J.A., Jones, H.E. and Kolodny, R.L. 1973 'A model for stages of group development in social work groups' in *Explorations in Groups*, S. Berenstein ed., Charles Rivers Books, Boston

Gersie, A. 1997 *Reflections in Therapeutic Storymaking: The use of stories in groups*, Jessica Kingsley Publishing, London

Getzch, G. 1988 'Teaching group work through reflection-in-action', in *Roots and Frontiers on Social Group Work*, M. Leiderman, M.L. Bimbaum and B. Dazzo eds, Haworth Press, New York

Giddens, A. 1991 *Modernity and Self-identity: Self and society in the late modern age*, Polity Press, Blackwell, Oxford

Glisson, C. 1987 'The group versus the individual as the unit of analysis in small group research', in *Research in Social Groupwork*, S.D. Rose and R.A. Feldman eds, Haworth Press, New York

Goffman, E. 1974 *Frame Analysis: An essay in the organization of experience*, Harvard University Press, Cambridge, MA

Gould, S.J. 1988 *Time's Arrow, Time's Cycle*, Penguin, London

Hagen, N. 1983 'Managing conflict in all-women groups', in *Groupwork with Women/Groupwork with Men*, B.G. Reed and C.D. Garvin eds, Haworth Press, New York

Hall, R. 2001 'Pitfalls and challenges in work with men who use violence against their partners', in *Working with Men in the Human Services,* B. Pease and P. Camilleri eds, Allen & Unwin, Sydney

Hanson, J.C., Warner, R.W. and Smith, E.J. 1980 *Group Counselling: Theory and process,* 2nd edn, Houghton Mifflin Co., Boston

Hogan, D. and Owen, D. 2000 'Social capital, active citizenship and political equality in Australia', in *Social Capital and Public Policy in Australia,* I. Winter ed., Australian Institute of Family Studies, Melbourne

Hornacek, C. 1977 'Anti-discriminatory consciousness-raising groups', in *For Men Against Sexism,* J. Snodgrass ed., Times Change Press, New York

Ife, J. 1997 *Rethinking Social Work: Towards critical perspectives,* Longman, Melbourne

Ivey, A.E., Pederson, P.B. and Ivey, M.B. 2001 *Intentional Counselling: A Microskills Approach,* Wadsworth/Thompson Learning, Belmont

Ixer, G. 1999 'There's no such thing as reflection', *British Journal of Social Work,* Vol. 29, pp. 513–27

Johnson, A.G. 1995 *The Blackwell Dictionary of Sociology: A user's guide to sociological language,* Blackwell, Cambridge, MA

Kahn, E.W. 1996 'Leadership gender issues in group psychotherapy', in *Women and Group Psychotherapy: Theory and practice,* B. DeChant ed., Guilford Press, New York

Kaplan, H. and Saddock, B. eds, 1971 *Comprehensive Group Psychotherapy,* Williams & Wilkins, Baltimore

Kelly, T.H. 1999 'Mutual aid groups with mentally ill older adults', *Social Work with Groups,* Vol. 21, No. 4, pp. 63–79

King, A.W. 1988 'Chinese painting and social group work', in *Roots and Frontiers on Social Group Work,* M. Leiderman, M.L. Bimbaum and B. Dazzo eds, Haworth Press, New York

Kurland, R. and Salmon, R. 1998 'Purpose: A misunderstood and misused keystone of group work practice', *Social Work with Groups,* Vol. 21, No. 3, pp. 5–17

Laird, J. 1995 'Family-centered practice in the postmodern era', *Families in Society,* Vol. 76, March, pp. 150–62

Leonard, P. 1997 *Postmodern Welfare: Reconstructing an emancipatory project*, Sage, London

Links Project 1996 *Increasing Access for Aboriginal People to Mainstream Health Services*, Western Adelaide Nunga Health Association, Adelaide

Long, S. 1992 *A Structural Analysis of Small Groups*, Routledge, London

Lyons, M. 2000 'Nonprofit organisations, social capital and social policy in Australia', in *Social Capital and Public Policy in Australia*, I. Winter ed., Australian Institute of Family Studies, Melbourne

McCallum, S. 1997 'Women as co-facilitators of groups for male sex offenders', *Social Work with Groups*, Vol. 20, No. 2, pp. 17–30

McGrath, J.E. and Berdahl, J.L. 1998 'Groups, technology and time: Use of computers for collaborative work', in *Theory and Research on Small Groups*, R.S. Tindale, L. Heath, J. Edwards, E.J. Posavac, F.B. Bryant, Y. Suarez-Balcazar, E. Henderson-King and J. Myers eds, Plenum Press, New York

McLachlan, G. and Reid, I. 1994 *Framing and Interpretation*, Melbourne University Press, Melbourne

McNamee, S. and Gergen, K.J. 1992 *Theory as Social Construction*, Sage, Newbury Park, CA

McTaggart, R. 1993 'Action research: Issues in theory and practice', *Annual Review of Social Sciences*, Deakin University, Geelong, pp. 19–45

Magen, R. 1995 'Practice with Groups', in *The Foundations of Social Work Practice*, C.H. Meyer and M.A. Mattaini eds, NASW Press, Washington, DC

Main, T. 1989 *The Ailment and Other Psychoanalytic Essays*, Free Association, London

Maines, D. 1993 'Narrative's moment and sociology's phenomena', *The Sociological Quarterly*, Vol. 34, No. 1, pp. 17–38

Manor, O. 2000 *Choosing a Groupwork Approach*, Jessica Kingsley, London

Middleman, R.R. and Goldberg, G. 1985 'Maybe it's a priest or a lady with a hat with a tree on it. Or is it a bumblebee?! Teaching groupworkers to see', in *Social Work with Groups*, Vol. 8, No. 1, Spring, pp. 3–15

Mondros, J.B. and Berman-Rossi, T. 1991 'The relevance of stages of group development theory to community organization practice', in *Social Action in Group Work*, A. Vinik and M. Levin eds, Haworth Press, New York

Mullaly, R.P. 1993 *Structural Social Work: Ideology, theory and practice*, McClelland, Toronto

Mullender, A. and Ward, D. 1991 'Empowerment through social action groupwork: The 'Self-Directed' Approach', in *Social Action in Group Work*, A. Vinik and M. Levin eds, Haworth Press, London

Neri, C. 2000 'Fabiana's change: How group psychotherapy works', *Bulletin of the Australian Association of Group Psychotherapists*, No. 18, November, pp. 42–52

Nosko, A. and Wallace, R. 1997 'Female/male co-leadership in groups', *Social Work with Groups*, Vol. 20, No. 2, pp. 3–16

Olarte, S.W. 1996 'Cross-cultural issues in group psychotherapy for women', in *Women and Group Psychotherapy: Theory and practice*, B. DeChant ed., Guilford Press, New York

Papell, C.L. 1997 'Thinking about thinking about group work: Thirty years later', *Social Work with Groups*, Vol. 20, No. 4, pp. 5–17

Parsons, R.J. 2001 'Specific practice strategies for empowerment-based practice with women: A study of two groups', *Affilia*, Vol. 16, No. 2, pp. 159–79

Paroissien, K. and Stewart, P. 2000 'Surviving lesbian abuse: Empowerment groups for education and support', *Women Against Violence*, No. 9, pp. 33–40

Parton, N. and Marshall, W. 1998 'Postmodernism and discourse approaches to social work', in *Social Work: Theories, issues and critical debates*, R. Adams, L. Dominelli and M. Payne eds, Macmillan, London

Pease, B. 1988 'Men's groups: contradictions, limitations and political potential', in *Social Groupwork Monograph*, Groupwork Unit, School of Social Work, Faculty of Professional Studies, University of New South Wales, Sydney

Pease, B. and Fook, J. eds 1999 *Transforming Social Work Practice: Postmodern critical perspectives*, Routledge, London

Pease, B. and Camilleri, P. eds 2001 *Working with Men in the Human Services*, Allen & Unwin, Sydney

Peled, E. and Davis, D. 1995 *Groupwork with Children of Battered Women: A practitioner's manual*, Sage, Thousand Oaks, CA

Petersen, R.D. 2000 'Definitions of a gang and its implications on public policy', *Journal of Criminal Justice*, Vol. 28, No. 2, pp. 142–50

Petronio, S., Ellmers, N., Giles, H. and Gallois, C. 1998 '(Mis)communicating across boundaries: Interpersonal and intergroup considerations', *Communications Research*, Vol. 25, No. 6, pp. 571–95

Plasse, B.R. 2000 'Components of engagement: Women in psycho-educational parenting skills group in substance abuse treatment', *Social Work with Groups*, Vol. 22, No. 4, pp. 33–50

Polombo, J. 1996 'Paradigms, metaphors and narratives: Stories we tell about development', *Journal of Analytic Social Work*, Vol. 3, Nos 2/3, pp. 31–59

Posluszny, D.M., Hyman, K.B. and Baum, A. 1998 'Group interventions in cancer: The benefits of social support and education on patient adjustment', in *Theory and Research on Small Groups*, R.S. Tindale, I. Heath, J. Edwards, E.J. Posovac, F.B. Bryant, Y. Suarez-Balcazar, E. Henderson-King and J. Myers eds, Plenum Press, New York

Putnam, R.D. 1995 'Bowling alone: America's declining social capital', *Journal of Democracy*, Vol. 6, pp. 65–78

——2001 *Bowling Alone*, Touchstone, New York

Quinn, T. 2000 'Challenging sexual violence: Social justice agendas in groupwork practice', *Women Against Violence*, No. 9, pp. 4–13

Rawlings, E. and Carter, D.G. 1977 *Psychotherapy for Women: Treatment for equality*, Charles Thomas, IL

Reed, B.G. and Garvin, C.D. eds 1983 *Groupwork with Women/ Groupwork with Men: An overview of gender issues in social group work practice*, Haworth Press, New York

Reed, B.G. and Garvin, C.D. 1996 'Feminist thought and group psychotherapy: Feminist principles in praxis', in *Women and Group Psychotherapy: Theory and practice*, B. DeChant ed., Guilford Press, New York

Rose, S.D. and Feldman, R.A. eds 1987 *Research in Social Groupwork*, Haworth Press, New York

Rosenberg, P. 1996 'Comparative leadership styles of male and female therapists', in *Women and Group Psychotherapy: Theory and practice*, B. DeChant ed., Guilford Press, New York

Ross, D. 1993 *Metaphor, Meaning and Cognition*, Peter Lang Publishing, New York

Roxburgh, T. and Domestic Violence Incest Resource Centre 1994 *Empowering Women After Violence: From struggle to strength*, Arena Publishing, Melbourne

Sachs, J. 1991 'Action and reflection in work with a group of homeless people', in *Social Action in Group Work*, A. Vinik and M. Levin eds, Haworth Press, London

Sapir, D. and Croker, C. 1977 *The Social Use of Metaphor*, University of Pennsylvania Press, Philadelphia

Schiller, L.Y. 1997 'Rethinking stages of development in women's groups: Implications for practice', *Social Work with Groups*, Vol. 20, No. 3, pp. 3–19

Schoener, G. and Luepker, E.T. 1996 'Boundaries in group therapy: Ethical and practical issues', in *Women and Group Psychotherapy: Theory and practice*, B. DeChant ed., Guilford Press, New York

Schoenholtz-Reed, J. 1996 'Sex-role issues: Mixed gender therapy groups as the treatment of choice', in *Women and Group Psychotherapy: Theory and practice*, B. DeChant ed., Guilford Press, New York

Schon, D.A. 1983 *The Reflective Practitioner*, Jossey-Bass, San Francisco

Schopler, J.H., Abell, M.D. and Galinsky, M.J. 1998 'Technology-based Groups: A review and conceptual framework for practice', *Social Work*, Vol. 43, No. 3, pp. 254–67

Scott, D. 1988 'Group work as a social network intervention', in *Social*

Group Work Monograph, School of Social Work, University of New South Wales, Sydney

Scott, D., Brady, S. and Glynn, P. 2001 'New mother groups as a social network intervention: Consumer and maternal and child health nurse perspectives', *Australian Journal of Advanced Nursing*, Vol. 18, No. 4, pp. 23–29

Shaw, M.E. 1981 *Group Dynamics: The psychology of small group behaviour*, 3rd edn, McGraw Hill, New York

Shaw, E., Bouris, A. and Pye, S. 1999 'A comprehensive approach: The family safety model with domestic violence', in *Challenging Silence: Innovative responses to sexual and domestic violence*, J. Beckenridge and L. Laing eds, Allen & Unwin, Sydney

Shulman, L. 1999 *The Skills of Helping Individuals, Families, Groups, and Communities*, Peacock, Hasca, IL

Spence, M.F. and Goldstein, B.P. 1995 'Managing the tensions between being task-centred and being anti-oppressive', *Groupwork*, Vol. 8, No. 2, pp. 205–16

Spiegel, D. and Spira, J. 1991 *Supportive–Expressive Group Therapy: A treatment manual of psychosocial intervention for women with recurrent breast cancer*, Psychosocial Treatment Laboratory, Stanford University School of Medicine, Stanford, CA

Spink, J.D. 2000 *Gender and Psychosocial Rehabilitation*, VICSERV Inc., Melbourne

Staub-Bernasconi, S. 1991 'Social action, empowerment and social work—an integrative theoretical framework for social work and social work with groups', in *Social Action in Group Work*, A. Vinik and M. Levin eds, Haworth Press, London

Stein, T. 1983 'An overview of men's groups', in *Groupwork with Women/Groupwork with Men: An Overview of Gender Issues in Social Group Work Practice*, B.G. Reed and C.D. Garvin eds, Haworth Press, New York

Sunderland, C.C. 1997/98 'Brief group therapy and the use of metaphor', *Groupwork*, Vol. 10, No. 2, pp. 126–41

Sullivan, E.V. 1984 *A Critical Psychology*, Plenum, New York

Sullivan, N. 1995 'Who owns the group? The role of worker control in the development of a group: a qualitative research study in practice', *Social Work with Groups*, Vol. 18, Nos 2/3, pp. 15–33

Taylor, C. and White, S. 2000 *Practising Reflexivity in Health and Welfare*, Open University Press, Buckingham

Thompson, N. 2000 *Theory and Practice in the Human Services*, Open University Press, Buckingham

Tiger, L. 1969 *Men in Groups*, Marion Boyars, New York

Tindale, R.S., Heath, L., Edwards, J., Posavac, E.J., Bryant, F.B., Suarez-Balcazar, Y., Henderson-King, E., Myers, J. eds 1998 *Theory and Research on Small Groups*, Plenum Press, New York

Toseland, D.W. and Rivas, R.F. 1998 *An Introduction to Group Work Practice*, 3rd edn, Allyn & Bacon, Needham Heights, MA

Touraine, A. 2000 *Can We Live Together?* Polity Press, Cambridge, UK

Tuckman, B. 1963 'Developmental Sequence in Small Groups', *Psychological Bulletin*, No. 63, pp. 384–99

Tudiver, F. and Talbot, Y. 1999 'Why don't men seek help? Family physicians' perspectives on help-seeking behaviour in men', *Journal of Family Practice*, Vol. 48, No. 1, pp. 47–52

Vinik, A. and Levin, M. eds 1991 *Social Action in Group Work*, Haworth Press, London

Wadsworth, Y. 1997 *Everyday Evaluation on the Run*, Allen & Unwin, Sydney

Walsh, J. 1994 'Gender differences in the social networks of persons with severe mental illness', *Affilia*, Vol. 9, No. 3, pp. 247–68

Warner, R. 1994 *Recovery from Schizophrenia*, 2nd edn, Routledge, New York

Weeks, W. 1988 'Feminist contributions to social group work practice', in *Social Groupwork Monograph*, Groupwork Unit, School of Social Work, Faculty of Professional Studies, University of New South Wales, Sydney

——1994 *Women Working Together: Lessons from women's services*, Longman Cheshire, Melbourne

Williams, W.C. 1976 'Pictures from Breughel (1962)' *Selected Poems*, C. Tomlinson ed., Penguin, Harmondsworth

Willie, C.V., Rieker, P.P., Kramer, B.M. and Brown, B.S. eds 1995 *Mental Health, Racism and Sexism*, University of Pittsburgh Press, Pittsburgh

Winter, I. 2000 ed. *Social Capital and Public Policy in Australia*, Australian Institute of Family Studies, Melbourne

Wright, F. and Gould, L.J. 1996 'Research on gender-linked aspects of group behaviour', in *Women and Group Psychotherapy: Theory and practice*, B. DeChant ed., Guilford Press, New York

Yalom, I.D. 1975 *The Theory and Practice of Group Psychotherapy*, 2nd edn, Basic Books, New York

Yalom, I. and Lieberman, M.A. 1974 'A study of encounter group casualties', in *Contemporary Readings in Psychopathology*, J. M. Neale, G. Davison and K.P. Price eds, Wiley & Sons, Toronto

Zastrow, C. 2001 *Social Work with Groups*, 2nd edn, Brooks/Cole, Pacific Grove, CA

INDEX

Printed and bound by CPI Group (UK) Ltd, Croydon, CR0 4YY

23/10/2024

01777665-0002